Pathways through Long-Term Health Conditions

Lifestyle Medicine to Maximise Your Wellbeing

Donald Moss
and
Angele McGrady

Pathways through Long-Term Health Conditions

Lifestyle Medicine to Maximise Your Wellbeing

© Pavilion Publishing & Media

The authors have asserted their rights in accordance with the Copyright, Designs and Patents Act (1988) to be identified as the authors of this work.

Published by:

Pavilion Publishing and Media Ltd
Blue Sky Offices, 25 Cecil Pashley Way, Shoreham by Sea,
West Sussex, BN43 5FF

Tel: +44 (0)1273 434943
Email: info@pavpub.com
Web: www.pavpub.com

Published 2025

All rights reserved. No part of this publication may be reproduced, stored in a retrieval system, or transmitted in any form or by any means, electronic, mechanical, photocopying, recording or otherwise, without prior permission in writing of the publisher and the copyright owners.

A catalogue record for this book is available from the British Library.

ISBN: 978-1-803884-23-3

Pavilion Publishing and Media is a leading publisher of books, training materials and digital content in mental health, social care and allied fields. Pavilion and its imprints offer must-have knowledge and innovative learning solutions underpinned by sound research and professional values.

Authors: Donald Moss and Angele McGrady
Cover design: Emma Dawe, Pavilion Publishing and Media Ltd
Page layout and typesetting: Emma Dawe, Pavilion Publishing and Media Ltd
Printing: Independent Publishers Group (IPG)

Praise for this book

"This compassionate and deeply insightful book offers a powerful roadmap for navigating the complexities of living with long-term illness. Grounded in the authors' Pathways model – spanning physical, emotional, and spiritual levels – it provides readers with a structured yet flexible approach to healing when cure is not possible. With wisdom and warmth, the authors provide more than just information; they offer companionship and hope through every stage of the journey. A vital resource for patients, caregivers, and healthcare professionals alike."

Inna Khazan, Harvard Medical School

"The Pathways model is one of the most valuable tools for supporting overall well-being through the mind-body-science model. By implementing small, steady changes over time, both patients and practitioners can make meaningful progress in managing chronic conditions and improving daily outcomes, whether emotional, physical, or psychological. This book offers more than just information and resources – it provides hope for those navigating chronic conditions every day."

Kelli Hughart, Sweetwater Wellness Centre

Contents

Authors' introduction 1

Section One: The Pathways Model 3

    Chapter 1: Living fully with long-term health conditions 5

    Chapter 2: A mind-body-spirit approach to self-healing 11

    Chapter 3: Steps to wellbeing: the Pathways Model 21

Section Two: Pathways stories and common long-term
health conditions 35

    Chapter 4: Regaining control and making decisions on
health habits (type 2 diabetes) 37

    Chapter 5: Putting heredity into perspective (high blood
pressure and heart disease) 55

    Chapter 6: Embracing nature and recovering inner
peace (cancer) 79

    Chapter 7: Dealing with difficult relapses and setbacks
(headache) 97

    Chapter 8: Recovering from loss of control, shame, and
isolation (irritable bowel syndrome) 117

    Chapter 9: Managing pain, recovering activity, and
improving mood (osteoarthritis) 135

    Chapter 10: Coming out of the tunnel of despair (depression) 153

    Chapter 11: Mastering the terror of the unknown (anxiety) ... 175

    Chapter 12: Integrating the past and living fully in the
present (trauma/PTSD) 201

Section Three: More guidance on creating and following your personal Pathways 221

    Chapter 13: Completing your Pathways Assessment 223

    Chapter 14: Selecting Level One goals 239

    Chapter 15: Selecting Level Two goals 245

    Chapter 16: Selecting Level Three treatments and professionals 253

Appendix A: Instructions for self-care skills 265

Appendix B: Apps, YouTube videos, books, audio recordings, and websites for self-care and lifestyle change 289

Appendix C: Healing Pathways Worksheets 303

Authors' introduction

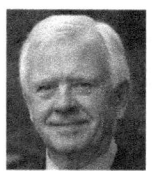

Dr Donald Moss is a clinical health psychologist and psychophysiologist. He is the Dean of the Graduate College of Integrative Medicine and Health Sciences at Saybrook University in Pasadena, California, USA. Moss's interest in integrative approaches to long-term illness began in his internship at the University of Pittsburgh 48 years ago. Over the decades since then, he has acquired skills in hypnosis, biofeedback, guided imagery, and lifestyle medicine in his mission to help human beings with persisting illnesses. His passion has been to help people with medical illnesses to help themselves, manage their illnesses, reduce their suffering, and live more fully despite their illness. He has published over a hundred book chapters and journal articles about various approaches to integrative mind-body-spirit healthcare.

Donald has many interests outside of work. He enjoys hiking, camping, bicycling, kayaking, gardening, and travel. In colder weather, he enjoys snowshoeing and Nordic skiing.

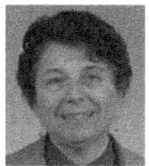

Dr Angele McGrady is a professor and clinical counselor at the University of Toledo Medical Center in Toledo, Ohio, USA. She has extensive experience in teaching medical, nursing, physician assistant, and graduate students the fundamentals of behavioral science. More recently, she has designed and implemented programs to prevent burnout and build resiliency in future healthcare providers. Her other interests are in performance enhancement for student athletes and the rapidly emerging area of lifestyle medicine. Dr McGrady's clinical practice focuses on applying the Pathways Model described in this book to the care of patients with complex long-term medical and emotional disorders. She has published over a hundred articles and book chapters.

Angele has many interests outside of work. She is an avid sports fan and loves to attend and watch college and professional events. She enjoys gardening outside and is proud of her inside plants, particularly her orchids and violets. Local theatre and outdoor music are favourite pastimes to share with friends.

Dr McGrady and Dr Moss earlier co-authored two books on the Pathways Model: *Pathways to Illness, Pathways to Health* (Springer, 2013), and *Integrative Pathways: Navigating chronic illness with a mind-body-spirit approach* (Springer, 2018). Both earlier books were written for a professional audience and contain highly technical, research-based examples of the application of the model. Though useful for healthcare professionals, Drs Moss and McGrady believe that the Pathways Model deserves a wider audience. They planned the current book for people who suffer from long-term illnesses.[1] Here they take a practical how-to, step-by-step approach to improving wellbeing. Although each chapter refers to a specific illness, the concepts of personal healing and regaining health apply to all patients with long-term illnesses. Readers will easily relate to the case examples, which are composites of real-life patients navigating their pathways to more healthy lifestyles and wellbeing.

For further reading

McGrady, A., & Moss, D. (2013). *Pathways to illness, pathways to health*. Springer.

McGrady, A., & Moss, D. (2018). *Integrative pathways: Navigating chronic illness with a mind-body-spirit approach*. Springer.

---

1 The publisher for the previous two books by Drs McGrady and Moss on the Pathways Model was Springer, and Springer has generously authorized the use of concepts from these books here to reach a wider audience.

Section One:
The Pathways Model

Section One introduces the Pathways Model for self-managing long-term health conditions. Chapter 1 defines long-term illness and explores the contribution of negative lifestyle and health-risk behaviors to the problem. The importance of modifying lifestyle and increasing positive self-care is highlighted. Chapter 1 also emphasizes the lived experience of long-term health conditions and the pathways to emotional healing.

Chapter 2 introduces several key concepts that provide the foundations of the Pathways Model, including the idea of mind-body science. The concepts are practical and will help you to manage your long-term illness, whether you are suffering from physical illness, emotional illness, or both.

Chapter 3 provides a detailed overview of the Pathways Model. It introduces the Pathways Assessment and guides you through goal setting in each of the three levels of the Pathways Model.

Chapter 1:
Living fully with long-term health conditions

Summary: Chapter 1 defines long-term illness and introduces the role of unhealthy lifestyle factors in causing and aggravating long-term health conditions. The chapter highlights the importance of modifying lifestyle and increasing positive self-care for long-term illness. The Pathways Model helps patients to effectively organize self-care activities, lifestyle change, and the mastery of coping skills, in combination with professional therapies. Patients are empowered to play a more active role in managing their conditions and improving their wellbeing. Following the Pathways Model also moderates the emotional impact of living with illness.

Keywords: long-term health conditions, long-term illness, Pathways Model, self-care, lifestyle change, quality of life, wellbeing

What is a long-term health condition?

The medical term for a persisting health problem is *chronic illness*. According to the Centers for Disease Control (CDC), a chronic illness is a health condition that lasts for one year or longer, requires ongoing medical attention, and limits or disrupts everyday functioning. Three chronic illnesses are the leading causes of death and disability today –

heart disease, diabetes, and cancer. Chronic illnesses are the largest factors driving up healthcare costs, with medical costs that continue for years, and personal discomfort and disability that can also continue for years. Chronic illnesses include all of the following:

- Alzheimer disease and dementia
- Anxiety disorders
- Arthritis
- Asthma
- Cancer
- Chronic obstructive pulmonary disease (COPD)
- Crohn's disease
- Cystic fibrosis
- Diabetes
- Heart disease
- HIV/AIDS
- Irritable bowel syndrome (IBS)
- Mood disorders (bipolar, cyclothymic and depression)
- Multiple sclerosis
- Post-traumatic stress disorder
- Seizure disorders
- Traumatic brain injury (TBI)

> *"...a chronic illness is a health condition that lasts for one year or longer, requires ongoing medical attention, and limits or disrupts everyday functioning."*

Some readers may be surprised to see cancer listed as a chronic illness, because common sense tends to equate such a diagnosis with death. Yet, as early identification of cancer improves, and as cancer therapies improve, many individuals with cancer live for ten years, twenty years, or longer. Cancer still requires ongoing monitoring and intermittent medical intervention, and cancer may continue to cause discomfort, pain, or disruption of everyday life. It therefore qualifies as a chronic illness under the CDC definition, and as a long-term health condition for the purposes of this book.

Long-term health conditions have one more thing in common: negative lifestyle and health-risk behaviors contribute to the onset of most of them and contribute to their worsening over time or erupting in "flares", or "episodes". Negative lifestyle factors that contribute substantially to long-term health conditions include:

- Sedentary lifestyle/inactivity
- Overweight and obesity
- Poor nutritional choices
- Social isolation
- Chronic stress
- Disturbed sleep
- Tobacco use
- Excessive alcohol use
- Chronic hypertension
- Chronic high cholesterol

> *"The good news is that positive changes in lifestyle can help you to manage your long-term condition and improve your quality of life."*

The good news is that positive changes in lifestyle can help you to manage your long-term condition and improve your quality of life. The Pathways Model is based on the power of lifestyle for positive health and wellbeing.

The Pathways Model for managing long-term illness and promoting higher wellbeing

Angele McGrady and Donald Moss introduced the Pathways Model in two textbooks for health professionals in 2013 and 2018. The Pathways Model provides a framework with three levels, enabling you to combine self-care, lifestyle changes, the mastery of new "self-regulation skills" such as meditation, with use of community resources and professional care. The Pathways Model enables you to become more active and engaged in your own healthcare, setting goals, eliminating behaviors that contribute to illness, and developing new behaviors that promote higher wellbeing.

In some cases, the Pathways Model simply allows the patient to reduce their pain and suffering, and improve everyday functioning and quality of life. Other times, the Pathways Model can seriously reverse some of the mechanisms of disease and improve your long-term health and survival.

> *"The Pathways Model enables you to become more active and engaged in your own healthcare, setting goals, eliminating behaviors that contribute to illness, and developing new behaviors that promote higher wellbeing."*

Self-managing an illness: an active role for you

What do we mean by "managing" a long-term illness? Human beings with long-term conditions function best when they become "active agents" in their own healthcare. This means reading about your condition and making well-informed decisions with your medical team about the choice of therapies. But it also means examining your personal behavior and lifestyle, identifying health-risk behaviors, such as poor sleep, that may contribute to your condition, and developing a plan to make better health-related choices.

> "Human beings with long-term conditions function best when they become 'active agents' in their own healthcare."

With long-term health conditions, a great deal of the actual care and decision making falls on the patients. One recent medical report concluded that patients with long-term illness generally manage their own condition and must make 99% of the day-to-day health-related decisions. Think about diabetes. Patients with diabetes monitor their dietary intake, record their blood-sugar levels, and adjust their diabetes medications when blood sugar is too high or too low. With today's advances in consumer medical technology, patients can do this monitoring effectively without sticking themselves to draw blood. Managing dietary intake and preventing weight gain also can play a major role in diabetes. Practicing stress-management techniques and relaxation skills can lower and stabilize blood sugar. Finally, patients must also decide for themselves when to request a medical visit.

Through the Pathways Model, you can set new goals to actively improve your wellbeing and reduce the impact of your long-term health condition. You can change everyday behaviors, modify your diet, activity, and lifestyle, and practice new, health-supporting skills, such as relaxation skills and meditation, resulting in a positive impact on your wellbeing. You can engage in spiritual practices, such as prayer and the reading of religious texts, or you can find spirituality in nature. All of these actions fall under the concept of illness self-management.

Building pathways to optimal health, even when living with a health condition

Common sense tells you that you go to the doctor to receive treatments that will remove a disease. People tend to think that pleasure in living and fulfilment with our life will return "when we get better". Living with a long-term health condition requires a new attitude and a new understanding. Effective medical intervention and effective self-care work together in long-term illness. The goal is to manage the illness so that symptoms are more moderate and less frequent. Knowing that long-term conditions are often lifelong, it becomes important to learn how you can live *with the condition* and discover quality in your life *while the condition continues*.

Our patients have taught us that even when they live with a long-term and terminal illness, knowing that their illnesses will probably bring death, they can experience the fullness of life – joy in loving, laughter at life's foibles, and satisfaction with their work, now, in this moment. The Pathways Model is not designed to cure every incurable disease, but rather to help you manage your long-term health condition and live fully.

The Pathways Model is based on an important discovery: the more active you become in managing your own condition, the better your quality of life will be.

> "The Pathways Model is based on an important discovery: the more active you become in managing your own condition, the better your quality of life will be."

Universal healing themes: the lived experience of illness

Human beings are not machines. Illness is both medical and emotional. We suffer physical symptoms in our body, and at the same time we experience deep emotional distress about the illness. The most common emotions for individuals with long-term conditions are anxiety, fear, depression and discouragement. Almost everyone with a long-term condition will occasionally experience anxiety about their condition and discouragement about the future. Yet the range of emotions that emerge around illness is vast. We may feel a loss of control of our bodies and our lives. We may feel angry at God or angry at ourselves for our condition. We may feel trapped and hopeless in a condition outside our control.

Whatever emotions you experience around your long-term health condition are important and are worthy of your time and attention. Medical research shows that illnesses are more severe, unstable, and difficult to treat when the patient is anxious or depressed. The Pathways Model invites patients to become more aware of their current emotions, feelings, and moods – the entire experiential side of the condition.

> *"Many of the self-care practices and lifestyle changes included in the Pathways approach can lift us from despair and re-awaken hope."*

Current research shows that negative emotions are not unhealthy. In fact, suppressing all negative feelings seems to increase the risk of serious illness. Experiencing negative feelings every moment is also damaging. For individuals with long-term conditions, it is not realistic to feel positive or happy every minute, yet long-term depression is also not necessary. Maintaining a healthy mix of positive and negative emotions is the goal of the Pathways Model. Many of the self-care practices and lifestyle changes included in the Pathways approach can lift us from despair and re-awaken hope. It is encouraging to take a very small step, by your own choice, and discover that it has a beneficial impact on your condition.

Final message: *Since the time of the biblical figure Job, human beings have struggled in their illnesses with universal themes, such as shame, isolation, a sense of loss, and anger. The Pathways approach invites increased self-awareness, acceptance of losses, and recovery of a sense of hope. A mixture of positive and negative emotions is the goal.*

Chapter 2:
A mind-body-spirit approach to self-healing

> **Summary:** Chapter 2 introduces important concepts that provide the foundation of the Pathways Model. The concepts draw on mind-body science, stress theory, lifestyle medicine, holistic health, spiritual perspectives, and complementary therapies. The chapter identifies the deeply personal nature of illness and the emergence of universal healing themes when human beings become positively engaged in their health. These concepts are practical and will guide you in managing your illness and improving your wellbeing.
>
> **Keywords:** long-term health conditions, long-term illness, Pathways Model, mind-body science, mind-body therapies, lifestyle medicine, physical activity, purpose and meaning, spirituality

The Pathways Model rests on conceptual foundations and medical evidence that have been developed over the past forty years. This chapter introduces concepts that will help you to understand long-term illness better and better appreciate the opportunity that you have to self-manage your condition. The Pathways Model is a mind-body-spirit approach to health and wellbeing that emphasizes:

- Mind-body science
- Mind-body therapies and practices
- Lifestyle changes
- Physical activity
- The mastery of new skills to reduce symptoms and promote the greatest possible wellbeing.

The Pathways Model recognizes that human beings are healthier when they have a sense of meaning and purpose, and when they can develop the spiritual dimensions of their lives.

Mind-body science

The mind-body connection is a two-way street. Everything that affects the mind affects the body, and everything that affects the body also affects the mind. Long-term illness is a perfect example of this principle. Stress can trigger or worsen an episode of a long-term health condition. But having a long-term health condition is also stressful and contributes to the total stress load in our emotions and physiology.

> *"The Pathways Model will help you design a personal self-management plan for your condition and integrate that with professional care."*

Long-term illness is a *mind-body problem*. Every long-term health condition has strong medical and emotional elements. Fibromyalgia, for example, causes pain in the musculature, as well as confusion, loss of attentiveness, and memory problems. This is why managing a long-term condition requires a coordinated team of medical and behavioral professionals and a program of well-planned self-management for the patient. The Pathways Model will help you design a personal self-management plan for your condition and integrate that with professional care.

Think about it. You may have a serious long-term health condition, such as lupus erythematosus, multiple sclerosis (MS), or diabetes. However, the symptoms of your condition are not always at the same level. In the case of lupus and MS, there are *flares*, times of much more serious symptoms and disability.

> *"Long-term health conditions are psychophysiological problems. They involve both mind and body, and mind-body treatment plans are needed to manage them."*

One of my patients with MS was able to chop firewood and carry it into the house on his best days, yet, on his worst days, his wife needed to call for help to lift him out of his chair. He did not have the muscle control to stand or walk. He also sometimes had full remission, with all signs of MS gone for weeks or months at a time.

Stress is one of the strongest factors bringing on periods of worse suffering with long-term conditions. People with diabetes often report that family conflict and other emotional stress seem to make their blood sugar more difficult to manage. Fears of possible job loss, a son or daughter's marital or financial problems, can all increase both the level of blood sugar and the lability (or changeability) of blood sugar.

Many other factors cause long-term conditions to wax and wane, to get more or less severe. Hormonal, inflammatory, neurochemical, lifestyle and emotional factors can all cause a flare or episode of long-term illness. Even the presence or absence of relationship support can affect the severity of both the condition and our suffering.

Have you ever noticed that nursing homes and assisted living facilities have many more residents who are widowed or otherwise single? Being alone, these residents lack the help needed to remain in the community and manage everyday challenges. Their long-term conditions are harder to manage, and placement in assisted living is the result. Long-term health conditions are psychophysiological problems. They involve both mind and body, and mind-body treatment plans are needed to manage them.

Mind-body therapies and practices

Many of my patients with long-term pain and long-term illness are angry when they are referred to a psychologist or other mental health provider. They often feel as if the physician is questioning the reality of their pain and suffering. My patients often angrily insist: "My problems are real. They are not imaginary. They are not in my head!"

Physicians refer patients to mental health providers for effective help with real medical problems. Medications and medical interventions can be helpful with some long-term conditions but are often not enough.

> *"The problem may not be in your head,
> but the solution may be!"*

Chronic pain is an example: the problem may not be in your head, but the solution may be! Patients begin to suffer pain for many reasons. Car accidents, falls, sports injuries, and ageing all can trigger the onset of pain. When pain is acute, lasting less than three months, it is usually the immediate short-term reaction to injuries. Rest, reduced activity, and analgesic medicine can often aid recovery. But over time, persisting pain becomes chronic pain. Rest is no longer helpful, and inactivity causes muscular atrophy and aggravates pain syndromes.

At this stage, behavioral health providers and physical therapists are often called in. Mind-body therapies, such as hypnosis, along with graduated exercise programs, assist patients in returning to a more active functional level. Hypnosis might start *in your head*, but it changes your physiology and aids you in tolerating activity. Many mind-body practices, such as meditation, muscle relaxation, and guided imagery can have similar effects, reducing the symptoms and pain of long-term illness. Mind-body treatments and mind-body practices provide a pathway for managing many long-term health conditions.

Lifestyle medicine

Physicians and wellness teachers have been recommending dietary and lifestyle changes for many decades. Patients are instructed to lose weight, stop smoking, increase exercise, and modify their diet. But making lifestyle changes is difficult and, on average, the world population is losing ground. Lifestyles are getting worse, not better, globally, and the number of human beings who are overweight and diabetic increases each year. According to the World Health Organization, forty-one million people die of long-term conditions each year, and lifestyle triggers the onset of long-term conditions and raises the risk of death.

In the 1990s, Dean Ornish was one of the first physicians to show that a comprehensive program of lifestyle changes can regularly moderate long-term conditions. Ornish's work led to the movement that we today call 'lifestyle medicine'. Our lifestyles can make us severely ill, but they can also assist us to better manage illness and improve our quality of life.

> *"Negative lifestyle contributes to the onset of long-term conditions. Positive lifestyle can help you to manage the illness, reduce symptoms and suffering, and even reverse some of the serious physiological changes caused by illness."*

For many of Dr Ornish's patients, lifestyle changes actually reversed some of the objective physiological issues caused by long-term heart disease. Dr Ornish organized a program involving whole foods, a plant-based (vegetarian) diet, stress management, yoga, and meditation for patients with heart disease. Initially, the program was residential. Patients had to leave home, take time off work, and enter an intensive residential program, which they lived 24-7.

Miraculously, his patients reduced their blood pressure, lowered their triglycerides and cholesterol, and restored better blood flow in arteries that were previously blocked. Angiograms showed that arteries that had been nearly closed by plaque formation were now open.

Later, Ornish modified the program to make it more accessible. Patients could participate part time, continuing their normal work schedules, and still show substantial benefits. Further research also showed that individuals with depression who completed Ornish's program also improved in mood. The Pathways Model is designed to help you bring about changes like this in an effective way, initially with changes you can make yourself.

Negative lifestyle contributes to the onset of long-term conditions. Positive lifestyle can help you to manage the illness, reduce symptoms and suffering, and even reverse some of the serious physiological changes caused by illness.

The role of physical activity

Being physically active decreases the risk of most long-term health conditions and promotes higher wellbeing. Inactivity or a sedentary lifestyle, on the other hand, contributes to weight gain, lower mood, diabetes, hypertension, heart disease, and cancer. The Centers for Disease Control tell us that a full 71% of the US adult population was overweight in 2016, and 39% qualified as obese. These numbers have been worsening each year.

Obesity and inactivity are a vicious cycle for ill health. When a human being gains weight, the drive to be active and the comfort with activity are lessened, and the less activity, the more weight gain. Further, self-consciousness and shame about body size can lead to avoidance of places where others might watch one's awkward efforts at exercise. Visiting a gym becomes torture.

> *"Being physically active decreases the risk of most long-term illnesses and promotes higher wellbeing. Inactivity or a sedentary lifestyle, on the other hand, contributes to weight gain, lower mood, diabetes, hypertension, heart disease, and cancer."*

For moderately obese people, even the simplest exercise can be physically challenging, and with severe or "morbid" obesity, joint pain and respiratory insufficiency often make exercise painful and even frightening.

In the Pathways Model, we begin with "movement", that is, increasing movement from the current level. Initially, this often means walking very short distances, and then gradually extending the movement for greater distances and longer times. Surprisingly, when our previously sedentary Pathways patients begin to walk short distances out of doors or engage in moving with music at home, they often express some pleasure and even joy at the experience. Including a child or pet in the movement can also make the experience more positive. Over time, Pathways patients can graduate from movement to exercise, and experience the positive increases in energy, physical sensations of wellbeing, and positive mood that come with extended activity.

The role of purpose and meaning

One of the first principles I learned in holistic health was this: *human beings who have something better to do don't get sick as much*. I saw this very clearly when I ran a research study on patients undergoing gastric and intestinal surgery for obesity. These surgeries frequently trigger a variety of symptoms, which are much worse for some patients than others. The symptoms are real and even life-threatening – especially severe diarrhoea, which can cause electrolyte imbalances and death. The adverse effects were real and had medical causes; the surgeries were designed to disrupt normal digestive processes, to cause weight loss.

> *"Human beings who have something better to do don't get sick as much."*

The nurses on the medical unit conducting follow-up were quick to tell me that patients who had careers they loved suffered much less severe symptoms and usually returned to full occupational and social lives much sooner. Patients who were unemployed or who had stressful and unpleasant work were often sick much longer and suffered more intensely. They were not malingering, to be clear, but they had no sense of urgent purpose helping to speed their recovery.

Our mind and nervous system work together to transform the body's response to illness, and our physical wellbeing changes. The autonomic nervous system modifies our stress response, with positive consequences. Muscle tension is lower, blood pressure is reduced, stomach distress lessens. Physical symptoms are moderated and feelings are more positive. That's right! Our *mental state* can govern and change our physiology, and this leads to improvement.

This same principle may apply to your long-term condition. Do you have activities – in work, volunteer activities in the community, and in relationships – from which you get joy and meaning? Or do you just tolerate your work and find life a drag and a burden? Finding something worth living for can be one more step in your Pathways Plan to moderate and manage a long-term condition.

Universal healing pathways and personal wellbeing

Illness is both a medical fact and an immediate, deeply personal experience. In the face of illness, human beings experience loss of control, threat to life, disruption of cherished activities, and isolation. Sometimes, illness provokes shame, embarrassment, and a sense of stigma. Religious people may feel abandoned by God, or may ruminate on what past sin might have provoked this episode of illness. These themes are universal, existential problems for human beings, not specific to any single illness.

Many of the self-care activities included in the Pathways Model, such as paced breathing, mindfulness, and journaling, facilitate enhanced self-awareness, acceptance of losses, and a recovery of a sense of hope. Through these steps, patients discover: "There are steps I can make as a person, and they can make a difference in my quality of life".

The case narratives in this book identify personal emotional and existential challenges, and introduce *universal healing pathways* that patients describe as they regain hope in their life and wellbeing. Regaining hope does not mean that long-term illness suddenly disappears. Many times, long-term health conditions wax and wane, and the patient's condition improves and then worsens. Amidst these waves of improvement and decline, human beings benefit from discovering their inner strengths, their resilience, and their acceptance of a life that is changed but is still a life. The universal healing pathways are visible in these moments of acceptance and hope. Appendix C in this book includes several worksheets designed to help people identify personal struggles and healing pathways to overcome them.

The role of spiritual practices and guidance

Dr Harold Koenig is a psychiatrist who directs the Duke University Center for the Study of Religion/Spirituality and Health. Two decades ago, he wrote that:

"Patients want to be seen and treated as a whole person, not as diseases. A whole person is someone whose being has physical, emotional, and spiritual dimensions. Ignoring any of these aspects of humanity leaves the person incomplete and may even interfere with healing."

In the last three decades, hundreds of research studies have shown that both organized religion and personal spiritual practices can have an enormous impact on our physical and emotional health. Persons who attend church services and engage in prayer and religious activities more often will, on average, recover from illness more quickly and suffer less. Religious activity has many beneficial effects, including social support and connecting with something beyond oneself. Many spiritual practices, such as silent prayer and meditation, also directly moderate the physiological stress response.

> *"Patients want to be seen and treated as a whole person, not as diseases. A whole person is someone whose being has physical, emotional, and spiritual dimensions."*
>
> (Dr Harold Koenig)

Yet people with faith and without faith still develop long-term illnesses and suffer from a variety of unhealthy habits and lifestyles. Occasionally, people with long-term health conditions believe that their illness is a punishment for some past sin. Such negative religious thoughts, shame, and guilt about being sinful, will contribute to making the individual suffer more. Kenneth Pargament, a researcher at Bowling Green State University, showed that negative religious thoughts create an increased risk of illness and death.

> "Setting spiritual goals is part of the Pathways Model. The goals must arise from the patient, from his or her traditions and beliefs."

In the Pathways Model, we believe in meeting human beings where they are, accepting their religious orientation, and drawing on whatever religious and spiritual practices they have developed, to help them with their illness. Setting spiritual goals is part of the Pathways Model. The goals must arise from the patient, from his or her traditions and beliefs. Examples of spiritual practices used by our Pathways patients include:

- Praying
- Reading a spiritual text
- Attending services
- Listening to religious songs
- Healing prayer circles
- Meditating
- Engaging in community service
- Pastoral counseling
- Walking on a beach
- Connecting with nature

For persons who lack a spiritual framework, and want more, it can be valuable to learn the basic skills of prayer and meditation. For some individuals, their personal Pathways plan can include meeting with an affirming pastor or spiritual counselor. Speaking with a spiritual guide or counselor can help you forgive yourself for any past actions and accept yourself in the present. Working through guilt and shame can be important for improving your medical and emotional wellbeing.

Final message: *Human beings are physical, emotional, and spiritual beings. Many mind-body self-care techniques can improve your quality of life while you live with a long-term health condition. Illness also often heightens spiritual needs and yearning. Setting spiritual goals and cultivating spiritual practices are helpful parts of the Pathways Model.*

Chapter 3:
Steps to wellbeing: the Pathways Model

Summary: The Pathways Model is an organized framework to help individuals like you plan and carry out changes in behavior that will moderate illness and improve wellbeing.

This chapter introduces and explains the Pathways Assessment and the three levels in the Pathways Model. The Pathways Assessment involves taking stock of your current problems and current strengths. Level One targets small, self-directed changes in diet, activity, coping strategies, and sleep. Level Two asks you to learn new skills – self-care skills, coping skills, emotional and physical practices, and encourages you to use community resources. Level Three guides you to combine self-directed change, skills practice, and professional healthcare. The chapter invites you to set goals at each level.

Keywords: Pathways Model, Pathways Assessment, Level One, Level Two, Level Three, self-care skills, community resources

Introduction

The Pathways Model helps people like you plan and implement changes in behavior and lifestyle that can moderate illness and promote wellness. We know that many small personal choices and behavioral changes contribute to the onset of long-term health conditions. A leader in lifestyle medicine, Dr Michael Sagner, identified nine risk factors that account for 90% of heart disease cases and a high percentage of other long-term conditions as well:

- Smoking
- Excessive alcohol use
- Physical inactivity
- Unhealthy diet
- Life stress
- Overweight
- High cholesterol
- Hypertension
- Diabetes

Making changes in one or more of these risk factors can help you manage your long-term health condition, and in some cases reverse some of the physical changes that it has caused. Remember Dr Dean Ornish's patients that were described in the last chapter? They made dietary changes, learned stress management, and practiced yoga and meditation. Many of them reduced their blood pressure, reduced their triglycerides, and opened up coronary arteries that had been closed with plaque. Lifestyle can make us ill, and even kill us, but positive lifestyle changes can restore wellbeing.

> *"Making changes in one or more of these risk factors can help you manage your long-term health condition, and in some cases reverse some of the physical changes that it has caused."*

The Pathways Model uses a three-level system to organize self-care into an effective way to combat long-term health conditions. We begin with small, easily achievable and self-directed changes based on your personal readiness for change. Instead of asking someone with a long-term condition to run five miles or spend two hours at the gym, we begin with walking to the mailbox or moving gently with music at home.

The value of the Pathways Model is that we cannot change everything at once. If lifestyle change were easy, you would not have purchased this book. Managing long-term conditions begins with small changes in our behavior, including goals you set yourself. Even small changes can have a surprisingly positive impact on your wellbeing. As you succeed with small changes, you will gain confidence for further and bigger changes.

> *"Managing long-term conditions begins with small changes in our behavior, including goals you set yourself. Even small changes can have a surprisingly positive impact on your wellbeing. As you succeed with small changes, you will gain confidence for further and bigger changes."*

We will introduce the three levels of the Pathways Model and encourage you to set some simple initial goals. Then, in later chapters, we will show in more detail how to apply the model for yourself by sharing stories of people who have used and benefitted from the Pathways program.

The Pathways journey: assessment

A Pathways Model Assessment involves taking stock of your current lifestyle, health-risk behaviors, emotional status, nutritional patterns, activity level, alcohol, tobacco, and drug use, social and relationship supports, spiritual resources, and other relevant factors. Only by facing your current problems and current strengths can you formulate realistic goals for a self-care plan. If you are currently spending your entire day sitting on the couch, setting a goal to walk five miles a day will fail.

The Pathways Assessment should also examine how active you are currently in managing your healthcare and to what extent you are ready for change. Many people are terribly frustrated and unhappy about their current illness and current life, yet are emotionally not ready to set and follow through on the simplest goal.

Factors to include in the Pathways Assessment are:

- Emotional wellbeing
- Cognitive wellbeing
- Physical wellbeing
- Nutritional wellbeing
- Substance use wellbeing
- Sleep wellbeing
- Social/relationship wellbeing
- Spiritual wellbeing
- Illness self-management
- Readiness for change

We discussed in Chapter 1 and Chapter 2 the types of strong emotions that almost everyone with a long-term condition will experience. Identifying your most prominent emotions, especially those triggered by your illness, is part of the Pathways Assessment. Once you have clearly identified prominent emotions, your Pathways Goals will help you toward emotional healing. We will return to the Pathways Assessment in Chapter 13, with more detailed instructions. We will also provide a graph that you can use for assessing each lifestyle area.

Level One: self-directed changes in behavior

Level One targets small changes in diet, activity, coping strategies, and sleep, that will restore your natural, healthy biological rhythms. Most people with long-term health conditions are overly sedentary, make poor dietary choices, and have terrible sleep. These factors disturb your body's healthy rhythms. In fibromyalgia, for example, most patients have irregular sleep patterns, which contribute to the mental symptoms of fibromyalgia such as confusion and memory problems.

> *"Level One targets small changes in diet, activity, coping strategies and sleep, that will restore your natural healthy biological rhythms."*

The Pathways Model asks you to assess what kinds of small changes you are ready to undertake now – not someday in the future, but *now*. Level One activities are simple and practical, and reflect your personal life experiences and choices. You might commit to using sleep hygiene principles to enhance the quality of your sleep, for example. You might commit to walking to a nearby park or to using calming music for self-soothing at the end of your workday. Or you may wish to commit to some small initial steps for changes in your food choices.

Level One: sample goals

- Paced slow breathing
- Dietary changes
- Improving sleep habits/sleep hygiene
- Walking short distances
- Moving with music
- Praying
- Sitting quietly
- Playing guitar or piano

You might engage in some simple self-care, such as taking fifteen minutes of quiet time in your bedroom or garden, or taking a hot bubble bath with some pleasant background music. Be sure to include some self-care practices that soothe you emotionally and help you manage the emotional side of long-term illness.

The magazine *Psychology Today* has some helpful positive suggestions for "true" self-care, which may help you identify target goals for yourself.[1] We suggest you choose two to three simple behavioral steps now, and then set a goal for when and how frequently you will engage in these chosen activities. We will return to goal setting for each Pathways Level in Section Three after you have learned more by reading the stories of others who have benefitted from the Pathways Model.

Level One goal setting:
Level One, goal 1:
Schedule:
Frequency:
Level One, goal 2:
Schedule:
Frequency:
Level One, goal 3:
Schedule:
Frequency:

---

1 www.psychologytoday.com/us/blog/changepower/202308/self-care-allthings-to-all-people (accessed September 2024)

A completed Level One goal-setting example:	
Level One, goal 1:	I will prepare carrots, celery, and other vegetables each weekend and snack on them after work.
Schedule:	I will spend time preparing vegetables every Sunday afternoon. I will snack on the vegetables from the time I get home at 3pm until dinner.
Frequency:	Snacking on vegetables at least three weekdays a week.

Once you have set some Level One goals, review them every weekend to see how well you have followed them. If you have not done well, adjust the goals and schedule to be more realistic for you. Choosing a more suitable goal can help you to feel that you are more of a success in your personal Pathways program.

Level Two: Acquiring self-care skills and using community resources

When you feel satisfied with yourself for setting realistic Level One goals and following them effectively for three or more weeks, consider whether you are ready to move ahead to Level Two. You may continue practicing your Level One goal/s indefinitely, while you move to Level Two. However, be realistic with yourself. If the combination of Level One and Level Two goals takes more time than you have available, discontinue one or more of the previous goals.

> *"Level Two in the Pathways Model asks you to learn new skills – self-care skills, coping skills, emotional and physical practices that improve your functioning and wellbeing."*

Level Two in the Pathways Model asks you to learn new skills – self-care skills, coping skills, and emotional and physical practices that improve your functioning and wellbeing. Level Two encourages you to use community resources and educational materials to support learning and lifestyle changes. Self-care skills include everything from learning paced, mindful breathing, to learning to pause before reacting, to keeping an emotional journal.

Level Two skills

- Mindful diaphragmatic breathing
- Progressive muscle relaxation
- Guided imagery
- Autogenic training
- Heart rate variability
- The pause
- Assertiveness: setting limits
- Mindfulness training
- Emotional journaling
- Meditation
- Prayer

You might use an educational CD or an app on your smartphone to learn to meditate. Alternatively, if you already know a meditation practice, you might set the goal of practicing the meditation at some specific time of day and place. You might attend a local yoga class. Progressive relaxation, autogenic training, and guided imagery are all basic self-care skills that you can learn using written handouts, educational CDs or DVDs, apps, and community-based classes. Heart rate variability (HRV) biofeedback is often a Level Three therapy guided by a trained professional. However, many individuals begin HRV training aided by a smartphone app or a handheld HRV device. Emotional journaling is simple to practice with the instructions in Appendices A and B, but if you learn about a journaling class, consider signing up. We can learn and grow in our emotions by hearing other human beings share their struggles and challenges.

Many of the coping skills and self-care skills at Level Two provide soothing and comfort for the painful emotional experience of living with a long-term health condition. Keeping an emotional journal, meditating three times a week, or practicing mindfulness as a coping skill, can all lead us toward emotional healing.

This book includes written instructions for learning several self-care skills, and a collection of web links for free online resources for learning self-care. You might begin Level Two by visiting the appendices of this book and selecting a relaxation technique you wish to learn on your own, such as mindful breathing or muscle relaxation. Look at Appendices A and B for instructions to guide you.

While this is a great place to start, many of us do better with live instruction. Have you taken stock of what is available in your community? Is there a nearby community organization that offers meditation classes or mindfulness classes? Are there 12-step groups that provide support and direction for individuals with addictive behaviors, such as alcohol, drug, gambling, or sex addiction? Is there a swimming pool that provides water-based exercise classes? Is there a local yoga studio that offers "gentle yoga" for people with long-term illness or physical limitations?

> *"Many of the coping skills and self-care skills at Level Two provide soothing and comfort for the painful emotional experience of living with a long-term health condition."*

Many online resources are also available. Dr Moss and his integrative medicine faculty have created a YouTube channel, called Saybrook University Self-Care. This channel provides over three hundred free videos, including more than forty excellent yoga classes for beginners and a variety of videos teaching mindful breathing, muscle relaxation, guided imagery, and several kinds of meditation.[2] The American Psychological Association also has a page of self-care tips, including instructions for how to do yoga from a chair if your mobility is restricted.[3]

Now, consider your current readiness, and set one or two initial Level Two goals. Be specific about where you will get the guidance for any new skills you will practice, and how often you will practice the skill. Remember, we will return to further goal setting for each Pathways Level in Section Three, so these goals are preliminary.

---

[2] www.youtube.com/channel/UCuPctVN1XIkyRE_W_bxvyWQ/videos (accessed September 2024)
[3] www.apaservices.org/practice/good-practice/Spring09-SelfCare.pdf (accessed September 2024)

Level Two goal setting:

Level Two, goal 1:	
Goal 1 guidance:	Where will you learn this skill? What resources will you use?
Goal 1 schedule and frequency:	When and how often will you practice?
Level Two, goal 2:	
Goal 2 guidance:	Where will you learn this skill? What resources will you use?
Goal 2 schedule and frequency:	When and how often will you practice?
Level Two, goal 3:	
Goal 3 guidance:	Where will you learn this skill? What resources will you use?
Goal 3 schedule and frequency:	When and how often will you practice?

A completed Level Two goal-setting example:

Level Two, goal 1:	I will take yoga classes and develop a regular yoga practice.
Goal 1 guidance:	I will attend the community centre 8am yoga class, before work, on Tuesdays and Thursdays.
Goal 1 schedule and frequency:	I will practice for thirty minutes after work and before making dinner, at least twice a week.

Now that you have set some Level Two goals, review your progress on Level Two activities each weekend, and if you are not progressing well, reset the goal, considering what you are ready to implement. Ambitious goals may be impressive, but only if you can successfully achieve them. Modest goals are usually more realistic.

Level Three: Combining self-directed change, skills practice, and professional healthcare

After you have practiced your Level Two goals successfully for two months or more, consider whether you are ready to move to Level Three. If you are unsure, consider staying with your current Level One and Two goals for another month, to really establish some new healthy lifestyle habits. You may also consider setting some new Level One or Level Two goals at any time if there is something else that interests you. One of our Pathways Model patients with chronic fibromyalgia was participating in aquatherapy, a water-based exercise program twice a week at a physical therapy program near her home. Each time she attended her aquatherapy class, she noticed a "gentle yoga" class meeting in the next room. After two months in aquatherapy, she decided to drop another Level Two goal so she would have time to do both aquatherapy and yoga. She continued these two activities for at least two years, as they contributed so much to toning her muscles and reducing her pain during movement.

Understanding Level Three

Level Three in the Pathways Model consists of professional interventions, services provided by a health practitioner, such as biofeedback, hypnosis, energy therapy, psychotherapy, physical therapy, acupuncture, or medication management. Most of our Pathways Model patients use at least two to three Level Three therapies during the same time period. When dealing with long-term conditions, synergy is a useful principle, which means that two or more forces working together have a larger effect. For many years, we have provided muscle biofeedback to patients with chronic pain, to assist them in relaxing persistingly tense muscles. However, patients frequently told us that they relaxed their muscles in the office yet tensed the same muscles again by the time they reached home. We discovered that if the patient also worked with physical therapy, together we produced better results. Physical therapists focused on muscle stretching, releasing trigger points in the muscles, and correcting misaligned posture. In this combination with PT, the biofeedback-assisted muscle relaxation had a more persisting effect.

> *"Level Three in the Pathways Model consists of professional interventions, services provided by a health practitioner, such as biofeedback, hypnosis, energy therapy, psychotherapy, physical therapy, acupuncture, or medication management."*

Choosing Level Three interventions

How will you know what form of professional intervention might benefit your condition? Consider your primary problem, your long-term illness or health condition. Are you currently receiving any medical care for this condition, from your primary care physician or a specialist? Consult that individual, and ask whether they believe that any additional therapies might help you to better manage your condition.

If your physician does not make any suggestions, do not give up. Many physicians are reluctant to recommend anything beyond the conventional medication-oriented care you are already receiving. Many of the optional therapies that might benefit you fall into the broad category of complementary therapies, and some physicians are uneasy about these options.

Common Level Three interventions include:

- Hypnosis
- Biofeedback and neurofeedback
- Psychotherapy
- Physical therapy
- Energy therapies (Reiki)
- Bodywork/somatic therapies
- Therapeutic massage
- Acupuncture
- Meditation trainers
- Spiritual counseling
- Psychiatric care
- Medical management

Complementary therapies are non-medical therapies that combine well with mainstream care and are increasingly integrated into an overall care program. Complementary therapies used to be highly controversial. The first federal program at the National Institutes of Health – the National Center for Complementary and Integrative Health (NCCIH) – was only founded in 1991 and was derogatively called the "Office of Unconventional Medical Practices". Today, however, complementary therapies are increasingly accepted and integrated into healthcare in academic integrative healthcare centres, such as the Osher Centers for Integrative Medicine at Harvard University, Vanderbilt University, Northwestern University, and other locations in the US and Sweden.

Is there a wellness centre in your community, or a holistic health clinic? Consider undergoing an assessment at one of these facilities to determine which non-mainstream therapies might benefit your condition and are available within driving distance. Ask any questions that you have including financial questions. Not all complementary therapies are covered by insurance, so cost may be a barrier.

Again, do not neglect any painful emotional experiences that are still troubling you, even after you have engaged in your Pathways Level One and Level Two activities. Healing troubled emotions is a universal element in learning to live with long-term health conditions. You might consider having lunch with a supportive friend or family member once a week, if you find that contact with this individual lifts your spirits. Your Level Three goals could include attending a local support group for individuals with long-term illness or beginning a counseling process. For example, Louisa, the patient with diabetes who is introduced in Chapter 4, felt stuck and was ready to give up on positive changes, until a counselor helped her and her husband discover the emotional basis for the family's resistance to her lifestyle changes.

> *"Healing troubled emotions is a universal element in learning to live with long-term health conditions."*

And now set yourself preliminary goals to add at least two Level Three interventions to your current healthcare plan.

Level Three goal Setting:

Level Three, goal 1:	
Goal 1 source:	Where will you receive this treatment?
Goal 1 resources:	What resources will I need?
Level Three, goal 2:	
Goal 2 source:	Where will you receive this treatment?
Goal 2 resources:	What resources will you need?
Level Three, goal 3:	
Goal 3 source:	Where will you receive this treatment?
Goal 3 resources:	What resources will you need?

A completed Level Three goal-setting example:

Level Three, Goal 1:	I will request a functional nutrition assessment and develop a modified food plan.
Goal 1 source:	I will schedule an evaluation with Dr Bell, a naturopathic physician with functional nutrition training.
Goal 1 resources:	I will use my health savings account to cover the cost of the initial assessment.

Can we skip a step on these Pathways Levels?

The Pathways Model is a framework designed to help people with long-term health conditions to organize a program of behavioral change, lifestyle modifications, and skill mastery, to better manage their conditions and achieve the best possible wellbeing. The Model is not carved in stone. If a woman finds a breast lump, she should visit her physician immediately (Level Three) and not spend three months making behavioral changes first. Similarly, we have assessed potential Pathways Model patients, identified a dangerous level of depression, and suggested starting psychotherapy (Level Three) and Level One activities at the same time.

Chapter 3: Steps to wellbeing: the Pathways Model

> *"The Pathways Model is a framework designed to help human beings with long-term health conditions to organize a program of behavioral change, lifestyle modifications, and skill mastery, to better manage their conditions and achieve the best possible wellbeing."*

In addition, most individuals following the Pathways Model will continue some of their Level One and Level Two activities long term, long after they have completed their Level Three professional services. The goal of the Pathways Model is to create exactly these kinds of beneficial, health-promoting, and long-term lifestyle changes.

In Section Two, we will share some case studies with you, to show you how people with several different long-term health conditions followed the Pathways Model, made long-term changes in their behavior and lifestyle, mastered new skills, added new therapies to their treatment program, and improved their health and wellbeing.

Final message: *The Pathways Model provides an organized framework for individuals with long-term illness to help themselves. The Pathways Model leads the individual through a self-assessment process, and guides goal setting at each of the three levels. Following the Pathways Model engages individuals more deeply with managing their health.*

Section Two:
Pathways stories and common long-term health conditions

Section Two tells the stories of nine individuals who used the Pathways Model to manage their long-term illness or health condition. Each of the individuals described here learned new self-care skills and made lifestyle adjustments. The overall objective for each person was to reduce behaviors and lifestyle elements that contribute to illness and increase behaviors that enhance wellbeing.

This section begins with individuals who exhibit the "Big Three" chronic illnesses: diabetes, cardiovascular disorders, and cancer. These are the most common long-term health conditions and are among the leading causes of death and disability. Next, we share stories of individuals dealing with headaches, irritable bowel syndrome, and arthritis of the hand. These disorders also affect millions of individuals worldwide; they frequently affect the individual's ability to live an active work and family life.

We also include stories of individuals living with long-term emotional/psychiatric conditions, including major depression, anxiety disorders, and post-traumatic stress disorder. Frequently, depression and anxiety are co-morbid with the physical conditions that we describe, that is, the patient suffers depression and anxiety intertwined with the long-term physical condition. Further, traumatic experiences in life, such as the early loss of a parent, physical abuse, or domestic violence, can leave people vulnerable to many long-term health conditions. The chapters on long-term emotional disorders describe people who struggle with emotional imbalance alone or in combination with pain and other physical symptoms.

The purpose of Section Two is to show the reader how the Pathways Model can be applied to a variety of long-term illnesses. The case narratives also illustrate a variety of options for self-care and lifestyle change for Levels One and Two, and the use of a variety of professional interventions for Level Three. After reading these narratives, we hope readers will be better prepared to develop and implement their own Pathways programs.

Chapter 4:
Regaining control and making decisions on health habits (type 2 diabetes)

Summary: Healthcare providers frequently hear patients remark that their condition has robbed them of personal control. They are locked into a complicated regimen, which they are told to follow every day. The treatment plan is presented to them with little opportunity for discussion about the practical aspects and the cost of keeping to the plan. This chapter uses Type 2 Diabetes Mellitus as an example of the specific challenges that chronic illness presents to decision making and the sense of control over one's life. It introduces Louisa, a 43-year-old married woman of Spanish origin whose diagnosis of diabetes brought on feelings of fear, inadequacy, anxiety, and perceived helplessness. The chapter explains in detail how Louisa used her Pathways program to make a series of choices at Levels One and Two, slowly increasing activity, improving nutrition, and learning basic stress-management skills. These changes created tension in her marriage at the same time that conflict emerged from her family of origin. Level Three interventions helped Louisa resolve these difficult issues. The Pathways Model helped Louisa overcome her fear, regain a sense of control, and make decisions for her wellbeing without sacrificing her marriage, her job, or her friendships.

Keywords: Diabetes Mellitus, Pathways Model, loss of control, dietary change, lifestyle, mindfulness, counseling

Healing theme: illness and the response to illness can disrupt family life

Sometimes, the diagnosis of a long-term health condition, such as Type 2 diabetes, though not life-threatening, creates a cascade of events that affect a very important part of a person's life. In this chapter, long-time patterns of food choices, meal preparation, and shared family dinners were upended. Lifestyle modifications, very reasonable in the provider's opinion, were recommended to a patient, but the same behavioral changes were perceived by the patient and family as extreme and drastic. Patients' decisions to slowly change their eating habits to attain better health may challenge the established patterns of the immediate family, extended family, and friendships. In this chapter, Louisa's diagnosis of Type 2 diabetes and her intent to improve her blood glucose control led to an unexpected crisis. Through the Pathways Model, Louisa was gently guided through the Level One interventions and began to notice some improvements in her condition. During Level Two, a surprising challenge arose from Louisa's husband. Through the efforts of the providers in Level Two and Level Three, the underlying issues were illuminated, and stability was returned to the family. Once again, Louisa was back on track and completed her Pathways journey.

> *"Sometimes the diagnosis of a long-term health condition, though not life-threatening, creates a cascade of events that affect a very important part of a person's life."*

Understanding Type 2 Diabetes Mellitus

Type 2 diabetes is a disorder of metabolism characterized by high blood glucose (hyperglycemia) and insulin resistance. The body may produce enough insulin to handle the food load, but the cell membranes have developed *resistance*, specifically, difficulty in using insulin to allow glucose to pass into the cells. Blood glucose levels increase. Patients notice that when they prick their fingers to obtain a reading with their glucometers, the results vary widely. Therefore, the diagnosis of Type 2 Diabetes Mellitus depends heavily on a venous blood test – glycosylated haemoglobin (HbA1c), which indicates average blood glucose for the past three months.

Traditional treatment for diabetes begins with education, usually offered by a diabetes educator who encourages lifestyle changes, specifically addressing better food choices and increased activity. Medical management begins with one oral medication, and then increasing dosages of the same medicine. Ultimately, combinations of oral medication and injectable insulin are the mainstays of medical management.

Less frequently considered by medical practitioners in a comprehensive care plan are the effects of long-term stress and negative emotions on blood glucose. The reader may recall that the classic stress response includes not only increased blood pressure and faster breathing but also a release of glucose from glycogen stored in the liver. In response to physical stress, such as running, lifting, walking rapidly, and biking, this glucose release is appropriate and necessary so that the muscles have sufficient energy to move. In contrast, under emotionally stressful conditions, the muscles are not using glucose and it therefore accumulates in the bloodstream. Negative feelings, particularly depressed mood and anxiety, are also correlated with higher blood glucose. Anxiety mirrors the stress response in increasing the release of glucose. The physiological association between depression and blood glucose is more complex, but basically, the shared path is through chronic inflammation. Behaviorally, both anxiety and low mood affect a person's motivation and desire to follow through on their commitment to change.

Introducing Louisa

Three years ago, Louisa began to experience symptoms of high blood sugar, particularly thirst, more frequent urination, and fatigue. At her annual checkup, her physician ordered blood testing and glucose tolerance testing, which resulted in a clear diagnosis of Type 2 diabetes. Her A1C value was 8.2% (higher than the normal of 6%). The physician prescribed metformin to be started immediately and also referred Louisa to a diabetes educator. The education sessions were delivered in a group format and emphasized diet and nutrition. The recommendations seemed drastic to Louisa. She was the usual cook for the family, but her husband, Leonardo, also prepared meals. They used recipes handed down from their parents and grandparents in Spain. Both took great pride in preparing dinners, especially at holiday time, for their two sons and Louisa's sisters and their families. Their reputation was unparalleled in the family!

When Louisa came home with the information about dietary changes, Leonardo was shocked. He stated that Louisa was too young to have diabetes, considering that there was no known history of diabetes in the family. Most of their knowledge came from stories shared by older friends who were on insulin. They frequently voiced fears of blindness or told frightening stories about low blood glucose. Leonardo stated: "How can we host the upcoming holidays for the family? We might as well throw out everything in the freezer! You can't have any of the wine I made for the holidays." Louisa burst into tears and left the room. There was no dinner that night.

There were other situations in Louisa's life where she felt that decisions were being made for her. She had a demanding boss at her data-entry job and was given no input into her schedule. Expectations were high and tolerance for mistakes was low. The office was noisy, which made it difficult to concentrate. But Louisa got along well with her co-workers who often compared recipes and boasted of bountiful family dinners. Several of her closest work friends were overweight and very sensitive about their shape and their weight. Mentions of weight loss or dieting were usually met with silence.

Family relationships were important to both Louisa and Leonardo. Unfortunately, Louisa's close relationship with her sisters had recently run into difficulty. One of her sisters had become very critical of Louisa and Leonardo's twenty-one-year-old son, Rafe, who was dating a thirty-year-old mixed race woman. Communication between Louisa and her sister, usually almost daily, had dwindled to weekly. This was hurtful to Louisa who had tried to talk to her sister about the diabetes diagnosis but had been rebuffed, as conversations came back to the topic of Rafe "disgracing the family".

The Pathways journey: assessment

Six months after her diagnosis of Type 2 diabetes, Louisa had made little progress. Tension at home, with family, and at work had worsened. Her productivity on the job had decreased and the demands increased. The holiday season had come and gone. The traditional dishes had been prepared and served, but the usual joy of eating together was absent. Rafe brought his girlfriend, so Louisa's sister refused to attend the gathering. There was tension during the meal. Louisa stated to her close friend: "I am trapped. My blood glucose has not improved. I am more afraid each day of the long-term consequences of diabetes, but I don't feel that I have any control. I am not in control at home, nor of my health, and for sure, not at my job. I feel abandoned by my sister and Leonardo is not supportive." Louisa's friend suggested that she request a one-on-one appointment with the diabetes educator who had been trained in a program called Pathways.

The educator was warm and welcoming to Louisa. She explained the Pathways Model and asked Louisa to complete an assessment of her wellbeing in ten areas.

> **Note to the reader**
>
> We recommend that you record your personal scores on the assessments listed below – as Louisa did, and as further described in Chapter 13. You may copy the worksheet from Chapter 13 or create your own record form. Use a five-point scale with one indicating very low wellbeing in an assessment area, and five indicating very high wellbeing in an area.
>
> - Emotional wellbeing
> - Cognitive wellbeing
> - Physical wellbeing
> - Nutritional wellbeing
> - Substance use wellbeing
> - Sleep wellbeing
> - Social/relationship wellbeing
> - Spiritual wellbeing
> - Illness self-management
> - Readiness for change

Louisa's self-evaluations were as follows:

Emotional wellbeing: Louisa experienced moderate to severe anxiety and her mood had worsened during the past six months. She worried daily about her blood glucose values and her diet, yet felt helpless to make changes. She was not happy at home, on the job, or with her family; she wondered how all this could have resulted from the diagnosis of Type 2 diabetes. She rated herself a *two* on a five-point scale for emotional wellbeing.

Cognitive wellbeing: Louisa was a college graduate and had finished with a degree in history with honours. She was confident in her cognitive abilities, though she admitted that her work performance had recently suffered because of her anxiety. Nonetheless, she rated herself a *four* on a five-point scale for cognitive wellbeing.

Physical wellbeing: Louisa's activity level was low. Her job was sedentary and when she got home, she was too tired to go out again. She had enjoyed long walks in the past and still got out at weekends. However, her motivation was low and the walks did not have the calming or restorative effects as they did in the past. She rated herself as a *two* on activity.

Nutritional wellbeing: Louisa told the diabetes educator that her nutrition was "terrible" and that she had "failed" herself, and was a disappointment to her physician. The perceived required changes in her diet were "impossible". Leonardo complained when Louisa tried to decrease carbohydrates in their diet and also stated that low-fat options tasted bad and were "an insult" to their heritage. She rated herself a *one* in nutrition.

Substance use wellbeing: Louisa enjoyed a glass of wine at weekends. She did not smoke, nor use recreational drugs. Her caffeine intake was two cups per day, well within the guidelines for the use of caffeine. She rated herself a *five* on substance use.

Sleep wellbeing: Louisa described herself as a night owl. She felt productive in the evening and stayed up late. The house got quiet, and in the past she had enjoyed the time alone, reading or watching a movie. Since her diagnosis, however, her sleep had been disrupted and non-restorative. The worry kept her from falling asleep and she was often still awake an hour after getting into bed. She awoke several times a night to use the bathroom. Sometimes, she couldn't go back to sleep, so went into the kitchen and ate a few cookies or a piece of cake. She was still feeling tired when the alarm went off at 6:30. She rated herself as a *two* on sleep quality.

Social/relationship wellbeing: Louisa became tearful when this topic came up. She asked to leave the session, but the diabetes educator was gentle and stated that there would be a plan to slowly make changes and Louisa, not the educator, would decide what area to work on. She also told Louisa that there might be other resources available. They would set goals in every area, but one at a time. Louisa stayed in the session but refused further conversation on this topic. Her self-rating on social and relationship wellbeing was *one*.

Spiritual wellbeing: Louisa was raised Catholic and continued to practice her faith. She attended services with Leonardo almost every week. Sometimes, the boys went with them. The family said a prayer before dinner and Louisa prayed daily. She stated that some days "my faith is the only thing that gives me hope that I can get out of my current gloom". She rated herself as a four to five on spiritual wellbeing.

Self-management and readiness for change: Louisa described her previous life, before the diagnosis of diabetes, as happy and fulfilled. She felt that her marriage was solid and their sons had not got into any serious trouble. They were financially stable. They saw family and friends often and shared many happy meals. They were people of faith and believed that God had blessed them. Now, her life had fallen apart. She did not know how to make the changes necessary to control her diabetes without disrupting her marriage and her relationships. She wanted to have her old life back, but could not reconcile the past and the present. She stated: "I am willing to work at this, but I am so scared". She rated herself as a *"scared three"* on readiness for change and as a *two* on illness self-management.

Louisa's overall assessment is displayed in Figure 4.1, showing the ten areas in the Pathways Assessment.

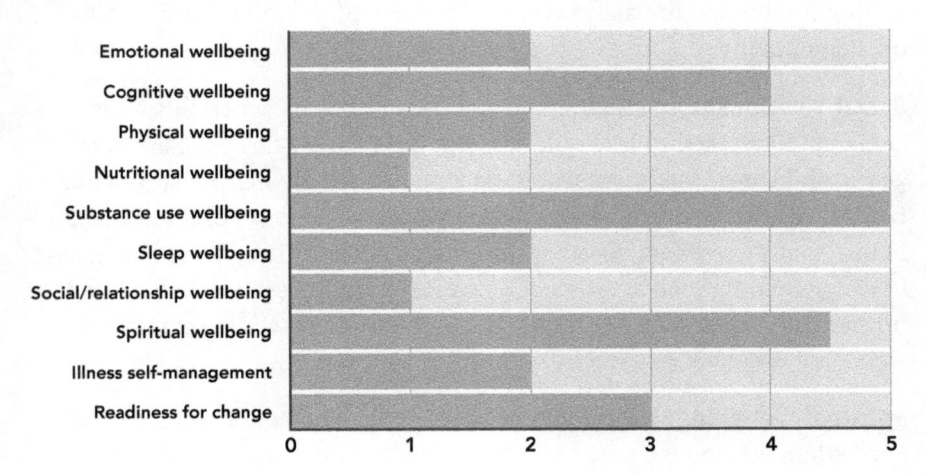

Chapter 4: Regaining control and making decisions on health habits (type 2 diabetes)

Figure 4.1: Louisa's initial Pathways self-assessment

Category	Score
Emotional wellbeing	2
Cognitive wellbeing	4
Physical wellbeing	2
Nutritional wellbeing	1
Substance use wellbeing	5
Sleep wellbeing	2
Social/relationship wellbeing	2
Spiritual wellbeing	4.5
Illness self-management	0
Readiness for change	3

Pathways treatment

Level One goals

Level One involves setting goals for self-directed changes, including self-care practices and simple lifestyle changes. Louisa's goals were around paced breathing, sleep, and nutrition.

Level One goal: breathing

A paced breathing exercise was the first Level One intervention introduced. Before practicing it, Louisa and the diabetes educator each counted their breaths for one minute. Louisa's resting breath rate was 14, higher than an ideal rate when a person is sitting quietly. Slow, paced breathing consists of inhaling for five seconds, holding for two, and exhaling for six seconds. The educator's voice was soothing. Louisa followed along for two minutes, took a break, then they breathed together for five more minutes. Louisa stated that she felt quieter and more peaceful. Her breath rate dropped to nine breaths a minute.

> *"Level One involves setting goals for self-directed changes, including self-care practices and simple lifestyle changes. Louisa's goals were paced breathing, sleep, and nutrition."*

Level One goal: sleep

The educator was aware of Louisa's frequent negative self-talk and her self-rated readiness of "a scared three". Even though Louisa's sleep patterns were unhealthy in several respects, the educator considered that too much information or any implied criticism would frighten Louisa and she would not return. She began by having Louisa recall a time when she enjoyed her hour alone before bed and when her sleep was restorative. Before the diabetes diagnosis, there were only "normal worries" – about the boys' report cards, friend groups, or concerns about work productivity, for example. After the diagnosis, Louisa worried about her health, her inability to make changes, the arguments with Leonardo, and, as she said, "too many things to list".

What had changed? Worries about the past day and what she had eaten that day filled the hour before bed and prevented Louisa from falling asleep. The educator recommended that Louisa use the breathing exercise several times during the day, during her hour before bedtime, and while in bed. Louisa was accustomed to praying at bedtime, so she believed that she could incorporate breathing exercises into her prayers.

Level One goal: nutrition

This was clearly the "hot topic". As described earlier in the chapter, cooking, meal preparation, and family dinners had become a battlefield between Louisa and her husband. Changes had to be gradual and realistic. The educator believed that the marital and family conflicts needed to be addressed by a Level Three professional but wanted Louisa to begin with smaller changes at Levels One and Two. She could control what she ate! Even if the foods prepared and served at dinner did not change by one ounce, Louisa had total control over her breakfast, her lunch, and her middle-of-the-night snacks. Louisa actually laughed as she stated, "Of course I do".

It was decided that the first change would be to stop the nighttime snacks, leading to a healthier appetite in the morning. Louisa stated spontaneously that she would modify her breakfast, which she usually ate alone. She would change the sugary cereal and toast to a bagel with low-fat cream cheese. She would add a piece of fruit. Louisa was enthusiastic about these changes, which surprised the educator, so she asked: "You seem so ready to change your breakfast – were you thinking about taking this step before?" Louisa laughed again and said, "Since I have been on the metformin, the sugary cereal tastes terrible, and I am hungry within an hour".

The next challenge was lunch during the working day. The educator reminded Louisa that she had full control over her lunchtime choices. "Ok, ok, I remember", said Louisa, "but my friends will notice and ask questions." Nonetheless, she developed healthy choices for lunch, which included hard-boiled eggs, low-fat cheese, fresh fruit, raw vegetables, peanut butter, and nuts. The educator provided a Healing Pathways Worksheet that considers attitudes towards nutrition and food choices. (Appendix C includes the Healing Pathways Worksheets for all chapters in the book.)

Level One progress

Louisa's worrying before and at bedtime continued to prevent her from falling asleep easily. Sleep onset time had decreased from one hour or more to about forty-five minutes, but awakenings continued. The hour of quiet before bedtime was still not calming enough. However, she used the breathing exercise at work and reported that she felt calmer during the hectic times when the office was noisy and deadlines were imminent. A few minutes of slow breathing helped her focus and improved efficiency. She implemented the change in her breakfast food choices with relative ease. She felt pleasantly full after breakfast and added a late-morning, low-sugar protein bar since her lunch time was not until 1pm. Others shared the same lunchtime and one of Louisa's co-workers asked her, "Where are the thick sandwiches of left-over roast beef that you used to bring?" For a moment, Louisa froze – thinking irrationally – "What if they tell Leonardo?" Quickly, Louisa answered, "The boys are eating everything, and I am left with dumb hard-boiled eggs". The moment passed.

Level Two goals

Level Two goals continue to emphasize self-care but draw more extensively on external assistance and community-based resources. Louisa's Level Two goals were focused on progressive muscle relaxation, mindfulness, and physical activity.

Part of the Pathways team included a behavioral specialist and Louisa's next appointment was with him. He reviewed Louisa's progress and complimented her on it, but she countered with a self-deprecating remark that her successes were only simple things. Her sleep had not improved greatly and the conflicts with her husband and her sisters had not changed at all. Then she added: "What if they find out that I am changing my diet?" The behavioral specialist had been alerted by the diabetes educator that there were deeper issues to be resolved by Louisa, but the main emphasis at this time was to build a sense of self-efficacy. He recommended continuing to focus on breakfast and lunch, which were going well. At dinner time, she could decrease her portions of high carbohydrate/high-sugar foods, and add an extra vegetable to fill up her plate. Louisa requested a weigh-in and was "horrified" to see that she had lost ten pounds. Then she spoke ruefully that since it was winter, and the weather was cold no one would notice.

> *"Level Two goals continue to emphasize self-care but draw more extensively on external assistance and community-based resources."*

Level Two goal: progressive muscle relaxation

Louisa's first Level Two intervention was progressive muscle relaxation. The behavioral specialist explained to Louisa that this exercise was specifically designed to increase her sense of control over her muscle tension and reactions to stress. This exercise can be done with the whole body (tensing and relaxing the upper, middle, and lower body muscles), or she could focus on one or two specific muscle areas. She could keep her eyes open and observe the tensing and relaxing or close her eyes. They practiced together, starting with a few minutes of slow breathing, and then going through the whole-body progressive muscle relaxation exercise. Louisa reported a significant decrease in muscle tension in her back, shoulders, and face. She kept her eyes open during the tensing and relaxing of the middle body (arms, abdomen, and back), and then her eyes closed naturally. The behavioral specialist recommended that Louisa use progressive muscle relaxation in the hour before bed, then use slow breathing and prayer when she got into bed.

Level Two goal: mindfulness

The next Level Two intervention was mindfulness meditation. Louisa questioned whether this was a religious practice, and the answer was no. Meditation is part of many religious traditions, but the application in this case was not religious. There would be no mention of God or a higher power. The objective was to exist in the present, experiencing the moment without judgment. When the specialist used the terminology of "blanking one's mind", he knew he had made a mistake. Louisa quickly said that empty minds invite bad thoughts and she refused to do the exercise. The emphasis shifted to informal meditation. The provider offered a cup of tea and guided Louisa in experiencing the sight of the pretty cup; the smell, heat, and taste of the tea. They sat in silence and drank the tea, and Louisa became less anxious and enjoyed the moment. Instructions were given to practice mindfulness while doing an activity, such as walking, eating, or observing nature. Since she ate breakfast alone, this could be an ideal time to be mindful and appreciate the appearance, taste, and smell of the food.

Level Two goal: physical activity

Louisa chose increased physical activity as her last Level Two intervention. However, Louisa cancelled the session that was to focus on physical activity. She left a message saying that she was grateful for the program, but she had to drop out. There had been a serious argument with Leonardo after their son Rafe remarked that his mother looked awesome since she had lost weight. Leonardo's reaction had frightened Louisa, not because she feared him, but because he was so upset that she *feared for him*. Something could be really wrong with Leonardo and Louisa did not know what it was.

Level Three goals

Level Three interventions involve professional medical, psychiatric, psychological, or other services and treatments.

Two weeks after the cancelled session, Louisa's diabetes educator, her original guide for the Pathways Model, reached out to her. She expressed concern and compassion and offered a brief meeting to see how she could help. Louisa reluctantly agreed but emphasized that she was dropping out of the Pathways program. The one-hour session was difficult. It was obvious now that Louisa had lost weight, but the provider did not comment on Louisa's appearance. The challenge was to re-engage Louisa in the program. It seemed that Leonardo had become distant, spending more time away from home. He stated that his boss had given him an important project that could affect the company's future. If this contract was awarded, then bonuses could be paid. At home, conversation was limited to practical things, with no real exchange of ideas. The boys noticed the change and were not comfortable around their parents. Louisa was used to talking with her sons about the day's events as she shared some of the more humorous things that happened at the office. Now, the boys left the table right after dinner and spent their evenings in their rooms.

> *"Level Three interventions involve professional medical, psychiatric, psychological, or other services and treatments."*

The provider encouraged Louisa, saying that something outside of her control, and not her fault, was affecting the family. "You and Leonardo have had a wonderful, stable marriage. The boys have never been in trouble. You are people of a deep faith. You have family and friends. You have a lot going for you. I admit that I don't understand what is happening. But I will do my absolute best to figure it out, but we need to continue to talk." Louisa thought for several minutes and then agreed, saying that she would continue for a few more weeks. She requested strategies she could use with her office mates about food choices and weight since, with the warmer weather, it was harder to hide her weight loss. She also asked for help with her sister, who continued to shun her family because she disapproved of Rafe's girlfriend. Louisa admitted to becoming sadder and sometimes being so sad that she cried before going up to bed.

Level Three goal: medication

Louisa's diabetes educator recommended that she consult with her general practitioner (primary care physician) about possible antidepressant medication. The doctor explained that even low doses of antidepressants help to lower blood glucose. She also explained that there is evidence that relaxation therapies are more effective in patients with Type 2 diabetes when their mood is more positive. This information was very surprising to Louisa. She trusted her doctor but also told herself that she would research these effects to make sure the physician was correct. (She never did this.) Prozac (fluoxetine), 10mg once daily, was started, then increased to 20mg after two weeks and well tolerated.

Level Three goal: counseling

The professional counselor specialized in therapy and stress management for patients with long-term health conditions. He evaluated Louisa and identified the major sources of stress as the diagnosis of diabetes, her husband's negative reaction to the diagnosis, the loss of a close relationship with her sister, and job stress. His conceptual framework was grief and loss of what she treasured. Louisa had lost her sense of personal health, her feelings of pride in preparing meals for the family, and her ability to confide in her sister. She was very hurt that Leonardo did not support her after the diagnosis of diabetes and seemed to be undermining her efforts to improve her health. The therapist agreed that Leonardo's actions did not make sense and supposed that there was a deeper problem, perhaps something from the past was frightening or angering Leonardo.

The therapist invited Leonardo to a session, stating that he (the therapist) needed some help because Louisa had become sad and depressed and needed her husband's support. After several weeks, he came, appearing upset from the beginning. The conversation was casual at first, as the therapist restated the strengths that the couple had as individuals, as a couple, as parents, and as people of faith. Then he gently prodded Leonardo to reveal his family history. Finally, Leonardo spoke:

> "There was a time when there were four of us kids and only Dad was working. Times were tough. My mother did her best to stretch out the food budget, but nutrition was sacrificed for foods that would fill us up. Us kids knew not to ask for seconds or to question why the refrigerator seemed empty. There was no subsidized school lunch program back then, so we carried our lunch, but it wasn't much. One Sunday dinner, my mother had on a loose-fitting blouse, which was lifted up by my younger sister. My father noticed that my mother was thin, and had no fat around her waist. He had a meltdown, threatened to leave the family because he was a failure – or maybe he should just kill himself since he couldn't take care of the people he loved. If he died, maybe relatives would come in and help. That was the worst day of my life. I was so scared. My sister thought she had done something terrible and was hysterical. My two brothers were also frightened and got up from the table. My mother told us kids to go to our rooms. She called her sister who lived close by and she and her husband came over.
>
> "After three hours of hiding in the bedroom and not being allowed to come out, my parents came to get us. They said that everything would be alright and no one was leaving the family. Life was not easy after that, but my mother got a part-time job and our finances improved. My dad suffered from depression, but never again threatened to take his life.

"Since that day, I was determined to provide for my family when I grew up. My wife and my kids would never be without enough food. I would never see my wife losing weight or my kids being hungry. I have never told anyone this story and I am sorry, Louisa, for keeping it from you. I knew that you were trying to improve your nutrition and keep your blood sugar under control, but your healthy actions connected to my terrors of the past. I love you so much; if the weight loss meant that you were sick, I could not take it. When Rafe commented that you were thinner and looked awesome, I 'lost my mind'. I went back in time and relived the awful moments of my childhood. I am sorry."

Louisa took Leonardo's hand as the tears ran down their cheeks. The therapist suggested that they sit in silence for a while, let the fear and angst lessen, and allow space for the healing energy to come into the room. They joined in prayer for peace and healing. Louisa and Leonardo attended four more sessions of therapy together. They continued to process the effects of Leonardo's past experiences on his perceptions of weight loss, and the thinner appearance of his wife. He spoke of Louisa's courage in continuing to improve her health despite the challenges of their heritage and his disapproval. He grew to appreciate Louisa's slimmer frame and healthier appearance and spoke about becoming more attracted to her.

Louisa continued in individual therapy for six more sessions. She needed help with maintaining her work friendships when co-workers noticed that she had lost weight. Specific dialogues were practiced so that Louisa could focus on her changes, without appearing to criticize her co-workers. At one session, Louisa laughed and said: "This is unreal; I am practicing sentences so I don't hurt the feelings of my co-workers – who should be happy for me – and who would be better off if they also lost some weight!"

The other major issue was her sister's reactions to Rafe's girlfriend and the distance that had grown between her and Louisa. This was a real loss, and grieving was therefore encouraged. Louisa processed her grief and eventually came to terms with the fact that her sister's behavior was partially a result of jealousy as she had no children of her own. She envied Louisa and Leonardo's family relationships and the way that other family members always wanted to share holiday dinners at their home. Louisa could try to re-engage with her sister but would always defend her son and his choice of a girlfriend as long as the girlfriend was a good person.

Progress on goals

Eighteen months after entering the Pathways program, Louisa had lost twenty pounds. She was proud of her A1C levels, which were in the normal range. She continued metformin, but slowly decreased, and then discontinued, the antidepressant. She continued to use most of the skills that she learned in the Pathways program, particularly progressive muscle relaxation, breathing exercises, and mindfulness.

Final Pathways assessment

Louisa repeated her Pathways self-assessments at the final session.

Emotional wellbeing: Louisa reported that her mood had improved, and her anxiety lessened during the Level Three counseling as a result of the individual sessions and those with Leonardo. She felt that the marriage was stable and loving again, and the boys now stayed at the table after dinner to discuss the day's events. There was much less tension in the home. She now rated her emotional wellbeing as a *four*.

Cognitive wellbeing: Cognitively she remained at a *four* level. Louisa believed that her job was not challenging enough but wanted to delay any major decisions until she was sure that her marriage was stable.

Physical wellbeing: Louisa rated herself at *three to four*. She had become more active during Level Two but had not progressed to the recommended minutes of exercise (150 minutes per week). She committed to continue to work on that goal.

Nutritional wellbeing: Louisa now proudly rated herself as a *four*. Her food choices had changed. She was eating more vegetables and fruits, and had decreased the amount fatty foods and sugary desserts in her diet. There was always plenty to eat, but the calorie counts had decreased.

Substance use wellbeing: Louisa again rated herself as a *five* in substance use wellbeing. She did not overuse or abuse any harmful substances.

Sleep wellbeing: Louisa rated herself as a *three to four*. Her multiple awakenings had decreased to one per night to use the bathroom. The time that it took her to go to sleep had decreased but still did not meet the recommended 30 minutes (from lying down in bed to falling sleep). She was still a night owl, so at weekends, she stayed up and then slept later the following mornings.

Social/relationship wellbeing: Louisa had begun the program at the *one* level. Now she rated herself as a *four*. Communication with Leonardo was very good and they had resumed their intimate relationship. She had spoken honestly with her friends at work and was surprised when they stated: "We want you around a long time, so do what you have to do to get healthy. We might get into Pathways one day." Louisa's sister was still distant and critical, but Louisa realized that she was not at fault for the deterioration of that relationship.

Spiritual wellbeing: Louisa rated herself again at a *four* to *five*. Her faith had sustained her during the difficult past months, and she would continue her attendance at church and her prayer life.

Readiness for change and illness self-management: Louisa perceived herself now as taking a high level of responsibility for her own health, reaching decisions, setting goals, and following through 90% of the time. She rated herself as a *four* in illness self-management. She also felt that she had proven her readiness for change, and she felt committed to further lifestyle changes. She rated herself as a *five* in readiness for change.

Figure 4.2: Louisa's final Pathways self-assessment

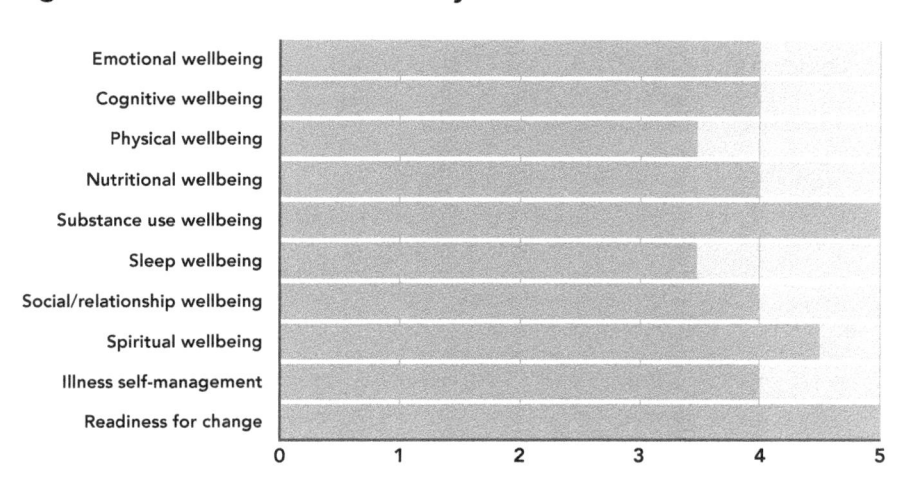

Conclusions

Developing a healing atmosphere, with little pressure on patients to make drastic changes is crucial to success. What appears to a professional as a minor, very reasonable and logical process may frighten or be threatening to a patient. Louisa returned to her Pathways wellness program after announcing that she was dropping out because the provider reached out, was compassionate, and created a non-judgmental atmosphere.

Recognizing and validating patients' strengths through the assessment process creates a positive framework for the work that is to be done. We must also recall that the patient who is in Pathways has others in their life who can be very influential and can affect the trajectory of the patient's progress. The healthcare providers must understand these other influences and the dynamic among the important people in the patient's life.

> **Final message:** *Long-term conditions and associated treatment requirements often take away patients' control over their own lives. The message to readers here is that by moving forward in a step-by-step fashion, with one small change at a time, you can regain control over your life. Paced breathing, relaxation skills, physical activity, and nutritional changes can all aid one in managing the distress that comes with long-term conditions. Further, counseling is sometimes necessary to help both the patient and the family explore fears about change.*

Resources

Diabetes UK. (2024). Diabetes: The basics. (2-minute video). Available at: www.diabetes.org.uk/diabetes-the-basics (accessed September 2024).

Goldstein, E., & Stahl,. B. (2015). *MBSR Every Day: Daily practices from the heart of mindfulness-based stress reduction*. New Harbinger Publications.

Learning about Diabetes. (2021). *About diabetes*. (Free informational booklets.) Available at: https://learningaboutdiabetes.org/programs-consumer/ (accessed September 2024).

Johns Hopkins Medicine. (2023). *Diabetes self-management patient education material*. (Free informational booklets and handouts.) Available at: www.hopkinsmedicine.org/general-internal-medicine/core-resources/patient-handouts (accessed September 2024).

National Institute of Diabetes and Digestive and Kidney Diseases. (2023). *What is diabetes?* Available at: www.niddk.nih.gov/health-information/diabetes/overview/what-is-diabetes (accessed September 2024).

Chapter 5:
Putting heredity into perspective (high blood pressure and heart disease)

Summary: Knowledge of one's personal heredity and health history is touted as important for health-related decision making. Young adults query older relatives about their life experiences, their habits, and their illnesses. Parents explain to teenagers leaving for college their health risks to give them an understanding of why they should avoid certain behaviors. When that information is not available, adults may rely on genetic testing to identify their potential risks. This knowledge is generally considered an advantage, and often summarized in genealogical data files for future generations. In contrast, information either given in passing, overheard, or mis-interpreted can create fear, conscious avoidance of medical providers, or a sense of impending doom.

This chapter describes the case of Andre, whose grandfather and father both died of cardiovascular diseases at relatively young ages. The religious service held for his father, DeAndre, emphasized God's will in life and death and was meant to give comfort to the family. Eleven-year-old Andre came away with a conviction that God can take anyone off the Earth at will, leaving spouses and children stranded.

Andre developed high blood pressure in his early thirties. He was advised to increase physical activity, lose weight, improve his nutrition, and was started on a low dose of antihypertensive medication. As Andre approached the age at which his father died, he became highly anxious and fearful about his health. His blood pressure continued to rise. He was referred to the Pathways program to consider what he could do to prevent an early death. During Pathways Levels One and Two, he improved his nutrition, increased physical activity and incorporated stress management, and mindfulness skills to manage physiological reactions to most stressors. But the belief that he could be "taken" at any time prevented further progress. Sessions with a spiritual adviser broke through the irrational fears of death. Finally, Andre put his heredity into perspective, became empowered to maintain healthy habits, and continued on his path to wellbeing.

Keywords: hypertension, Pathways Model, heredity, nutrition, stress management, healthy habits, beliefs, spiritual advising

Healing theme: heredity is not destiny

The healing theme of this chapter is integrating knowledge of inheritance and genetic factors into a comprehensive, logical approach to wellbeing. The strong history of cardiovascular disease on the paternal side of Andre's family was factual. Information about the tendency to inherit high blood pressure and heart disease combined with a minister's well-intended statements were heard by a young boy grieving for his father. As he aged into adulthood, Andre became obsessed with worry and a sense of impending doom. The belief that death could come through the actions of a higher power against which a mere human has no control became terrifying for him. Andre experienced a psychological roadblock that prevented him from taking sufficient action to decrease his health risk.

> *"The healing theme of this chapter is integrating knowledge of inheritance and genetic factors into a comprehensive, logical approach to wellbeing."*

Andre was an intelligent, educated accountant. He worked hard and was rewarded by moving up in the company to a supervisory position. In any analytic situation that affected his family, he was rational, clear minded, and logical; he did research before making decisions on such things as where to buy a home, where the kids should go to school and financial matters. But in the area of his own health, he believed that his heredity and God's plan for him overwhelmed any personal efforts. Andre wanted to live, to be there when his son grew up, in contrast to his own experience of losing his father at eleven. Andre entered the Pathways program to save his son from the same grief that he had experienced. The activities used in the Pathways Model Levels One and Two are backed up by extensive research, so Andre accepted the challenge to modify his diet, physical activity, and the ways that he managed stress. However, spiritual guidance was necessary for Andre to lessen the perceived burden of his heredity and instead integrate the knowledge of his family history into a plan to maintain his health and prevent heart disease.

Understanding essential (primary) hypertension

Primary hypertension indicates higher-than-normal blood pressure and is a very common chronic illness affecting the adult population. Blood pressure (BP) is defined as systolic and diastolic values, which are measured in millimetres of mercury. Systolic pressure – the first number – indicates the force of the blood against the walls of the artery when the heart contracts. The diastolic pressure – the second number – refers to the pressure that blood exerts against the artery walls when the heart is between beats.

The level of pressure needs to be sufficient to send blood to tissues close to and distant from the heart. Enough pressure is also needed to perfuse muscles when the person is active and to allow the brain to function while the person is awake. So, a mechanism must exist to vary blood pressure depending on the body's demands. In other words, increases in blood pressure are necessary for normal day-to-day function. During exercise, for example, BP increases to levels equivalent to hypertension; yet regular exercise is known to reduce blood pressure. When a person is excited while watching a movie, dancing, or engaged in intimacy, BP increases, and these activities are viewed as positive and enjoyable. Why is one

Chapter 5: Putting heredity into perspective (high blood pressure and heart disease)

circumstance healthy while the other is not? BP must be in a certain range at rest, and the changes during the activities listed above are relatively short lasting. Blood vessels are not damaged by short-term increases in BP.

Sustained elevated BP (hypertension) results from multiple factors. A person who is overweight, smokes, overuses alcohol, and/or eats a high-salt or fatty diet is definitely at risk for developing hypertension. In addition, stress has a major influence on the cardiovascular system, specifically increased BP, heart rate, and the constriction of blood vessels. Short-term stress is sometimes positive, for example, when the person is excited, faces a challenge, or receives good news. However, when stress becomes constant, the BP, heart rate, and breathing rate remain elevated and there is minimal recovery, or return to resting BP is slowed.

> *"A person who is overweight, smokes, overuses alcohol, and/or eats a high salt or fatty diet is definitely at risk for developing hypertension. In addition, stress has a major influence on the cardiovascular system, specifically increased BP, heart rate, and the constriction of blood vessels."*

The effects of stress overlap with other behaviors that have negative influences on the cardiovascular system. A person coping with financial problems or living in a crowded, noisy apartment becomes worried and anxious but doesn't have the relaxation or mindfulness tools to decrease the effects of stress. That person may not have access to healthy food options or may not feel safe walking in their neighbourhood. The person who becomes sad or depressed because they are criticized at work, or because they are going through a divorce, will not have restorative sleep and will be tired in the morning, rushing out the door without breakfast, and grabbing fast food on the way to work.

An accurate diagnosis of primary hypertension depends on measurements made under different conditions. BP is measured in the physician's office as part of a routine exam; ideally, several measurements are made in both arms while the person is sitting quietly. Home BP readings over a week or two are also important since some individuals will have elevated blood pressure in the doctor's office due to the stress of the situation. According to the International Society of Hypertension, the threshold BP for diagnosis is 140/90 mm Hg in the office and 135/85 mm Hg at home. The American College of Cardiology sets lower ranges for normal blood pressure, recommending treatment at a threshold of 130/80 mmHg. Both entities agree on the necessity of accurate measurements and the assessment of overall risk before beginning treatment.

> *"Lifestyle modifications are first level interventions, unless the person has multiple other risk factors, such as Type 2 diabetes or high cholesterol."*

Lifestyle modifications are first-level interventions, unless the person has multiple other risk factors, such as Type 2 diabetes or high cholesterol. In particular, diabetes confers additional risk because high blood sugar affects the health of the blood vessels and the heart. High blood levels of LDL (low-density lipoproteins) and overall cholesterol levels increase the risk of heart disease and stroke, due to the narrowing of the arteries.

The following lifestyle recommendations are based on reliable research evidence: increasing physical activity, lowering salt intake, decreasing alcohol use, stopping smoking, losing weight, and managing stress. The DASH diet (Dietary Approaches to Stop Hypertension) is one example of a nutritional plan which focuses on the reduction of salt intake, increasing fruits, vegetables, and high-quality foods, and decreasing consumption of sugar- and fat-laden foods and beverages. There are other approaches to improving nutrition, such as the Mediterranean diet, and the Healthy Eating Plate, but the basic principles are the same. Although the evidence supporting nutritional supplements or vitamins is not as robust, many can be safely tried. We recommend that readers consult the websites listed at the end of this chapter, and consult with a general practice physician, particularly to check on interactions between prescribed medication and supplements.

> *"The following lifestyle recommendations are based on reliable research evidence: increasing physical activity, lowering salt intake, decreasing alcohol use, stopping smoking, losing weight, and managing stress."*

Physical activity is a major component of lifestyle modification, particularly in individuals who are mostly sedentary. Gradual increases in aerobic activity (actions that involve moving the large muscles of the body in rhythm) are recommended with the goal of achieving 150 minutes of moderate-intensity activity per week. Strength training (actions in which the muscles do more work than they usually do) involves lifting weights and these are part of the 150 minutes of recommended activity. Again, we refer readers to the list of readings and websites at the end of this chapter; in addition, consultation with a general practice physician will ensure that it is safe to begin an exercise program.

> *"Physical activity is a major component of lifestyle modification, particularly in individuals who are mostly sedentary."*

Stress management has documented efficacy in reducing high BP, since relaxation decreases heart rate and increases dilation of the blood vessels. Breathing exercises, general relaxation, imagery, biofeedback, and mindfulness meditation are examples of stress-management interventions. It is also important to emphasize that making changes in one aspect of lifestyle often confers significant benefits to other components of lifestyle, similar to the previous examples of high stress creating less motivation to exercise or cook nutritional meals. For example, learning and using relaxation skills at bedtime allows a person to fall asleep more quickly and facilitates more restorative sleep. Awakening with more energy increases motivation to make time for breakfast and to plan for a healthy lunch and dinner.

> *"Stress management has documented efficacy in reducing high BP, since relaxation decreases heart rate and increases dilation of the blood vessels. Breathing exercises, general relaxation, imagery, biofeedback and mindfulness meditation are examples of stress management interventions."*

Medication is started when the person cannot implement or does not improve with lifestyle modifications within a three-to-six-month time frame. The four major classes of antihypertensive drugs are diuretics, beta blockers, calcium channel blockers, and renin angiotensin system inhibitors (including angiotensin-converting enzyme inhibitors and angiotensin receptor blockers). The prescribing physician may begin with a low dose of one drug and monitor the response. If the target BP is not reached, the dosage of the first medicine will be increased or a combination of drugs will be used. Monitoring continues in the office and home settings to confirm the benefit of both the lifestyle changes and medication.

> *"Medication is started when the person cannot implement or does not improve with lifestyle modifications within a three-to-six-month time frame."*

Introducing Andre

Andre was a forty-eight-year-old man who had been diagnosed with essential (primary) hypertension in his early thirties. Andre revealed his family history of stroke and heart attack to his medical provider. Specifically, his father, DeAndre, had died at age fifty of a haemorrhagic stroke, and his grandfather, DellAndre, had died of a heart attack when he was fifty-five years old.

Andre was a college graduate, the first in his family. He worked full time as a certified accountant in a large firm. His accounts were businesses

Chapter 5: Putting heredity into perspective (high blood pressure and heart disease)

and corporations, so he often travelled with his team to conduct audits at company headquarters. He was very skilled at his job and well respected in the company. He had recently been promoted to supervisor of four junior accountants. His colleagues described him as "logical, reasonable, and a real numbers man".

Andre was married to Winnie. Winnie worked as a receptionist in the same accounting firm. They had three children: two girls, aged eleven and eight, and a son, aged fifteen. Andre and Winnie carried on the tradition of names on Andre's side of the family and named their son Andrell. The children were healthy and active and did well in school.

Andre and Winnie had both been brought up in the Methodist church, had been confirmed, and attended services with their families. When Andre started college, he did not continue any of his religious practices. Winnie wished to be married in the Methodist church and Andre agreed. Their children were baptized, went to Sunday school, and regularly attended services with Winne. Andre was supportive of Winnie and the kids maintaining their connection with the church, but did not engage in conversations with anyone about his own religious beliefs.

Andre's grandfather, DellAndre, had been a farmer who worked long hours and came home exhausted at night. He had believed that one day in the week should be devoted to gatherings of family and friends, and Andre heard many stories about these events. It was said that the supply of homemade wine and beer was unending – sometimes guests spent the night because no one left DellAndre's home to drive home drunk. One day, DellAndre complained of chest pain, but told his wife that he had eaten too much the day before. During the night, the pain intensified, and he cried out. The ambulance was called, but by the time DellAndre arrived at the hospital, it was too late; he had died of a heart attack at age fifty-five.

Andre grew up with two sisters and both parents in the home. Although his father, DeAndre, only finished high school, he worked his way up to become a manager in a linen supply company. The family was able to afford yearly vacations and enjoyed their time together. Andre felt close to his dad and was proud to be named according to the family tradition. Andre and DeAndre shared several interests, particularly sports and local history. DeAndre had had high blood pressure for years and occasionally a family member would comment on his ruddy complexion. DeAndre's physician prescribed an antihypertensive medication, but DeAndre took the medicine only sporadically. He did not engage in any regular physical activity. DeAndre spoke sarcastically: "Going to the gym is for people who don't work in the linen business; I am on my feet all day!"

At age fifty, DeAndre had a stroke; he was at work at the time, so the emergency medical services were called. He lost function on his right side and also had difficulty speaking. He was sent home after a week in hospital to rehabilitate at home. It was a very stressful time for the family. The strong, successful family patriarch had trouble walking and communicating. He was often misunderstood and mixed up words. Andre was frightened when his father became angry out of frustration and yelled at his mother or at Andre and his sisters. He heard his father crying at night and his mother trying to soothe him. Their conversations about sports were fewer and fewer since DeAndre could not follow the flow of the games or fell asleep during critical periods of play. Eight weeks after the initial stroke, he had another stroke that was fatal.

DeAndre's religious services brought a large number of people to the church since he was popular in the community. The minister praised him liberally, and then attempted to put his early death into perspective for the mourners. He stated: "The death was God's will. God has a plan for everyone, and He took DeAndre because that was His plan for him." "No one can be guaranteed heaven," he commented but suggested that the congregation pray that DeAndre be "allowed into heaven". He reassured the congregation that "God will take care of the family".

Andre went over these words for weeks after his father's death. He repeatedly questioned his mother and asked, "How is God taking care of us?" His mother replied that God had inspired his dad to take out a life insurance policy that had been cashed in. God also made it possible for his mother to find a job which she loved. Further, Andre asked, "When will we know that Dad is in heaven and what if he isn't allowed in? Where is Dad if he is not in heaven?" There was no answer to this question, but his mother was sure that his dad was in heaven. Andre stated: "I wish God had left Dad on earth; maybe He could have taken someone else who didn't have kids instead of my dad". After many of these conversations, his mother hushed Andre and told him to accept God's will.

As the years went on, Andre could never forget the sermon that the minister had given. When he himself was diagnosed with high blood pressure at age thirty-three, his first reaction was intense fear, then anger. "This is the beginning of the end for me, and my kids will not have their father for much longer. I named my son in the family tradition, but maybe I have cursed him, instead of honouring our heritage. God knows Andre's family. God is going to take me and leave my son without his father."

Andre's physician recommended lifestyle modifications and wanted Andre to consider medication. Knowing Andre's need for evidence, he encouraged Andre to do research on nutrition, physical activity, and relaxation. The physician commented: "There is continuous progress in the field of hypertension and some of the interventions that I can offer were not available to your father, and certainly not to your grandfather. There are effective medicines and emerging research on supplements; there are mental exercises, like meditation, relaxation, and imagery."

Andre listened politely and agreed to take a low-dose antihypertensive medication. But he believed that "nothing can go against God's plan". He told his doctor, "Thank you for your care of me, but I am doomed, and it does not matter what I do". The physician was surprised by what Andre said. He queried Andre about thoughts of self-harm. Andre scoffed at this question. "Of course, I am not suicidal; I would never intentionally leave my family. But none of this is in my hands; there is a higher power who has taken my father and my grandfather off the earth, and I am next."

Andre exhibited early signs of heart disease, so the physician wanted him to accept a referral to a cardiologist. Considering the family history, the physician reasoned that Andre should be established with a specialist in case (the physician thought when) the hypertension worsened and started affecting the major arteries or his heart. Andre forcefully refused the referral to a cardiologist. He remembered his mother mentioning a special doctor for the heart when his father became ill, and he was terrified. He believed that the first appointment would be the beginning of the downward slide. "God will be waiting for His chance to take me," he thought.

> *"When Andre refused an increase in medicine, or a referral to a cardiologist, the physician told Andre that there was a program called Pathways, where Andre could learn to develop more of a sense of control over his blood pressure."*

When Andre refused an increase in medicine, or a referral to a cardiologist, the physician told Andre that there was a program called Pathways, where Andre could learn to develop more of a sense of control over his blood pressure. The idea of gaining control resonated with Andre, and he felt a glimmer of hope. He agreed to the referral.

The Pathways journey: assessment

Andre was encouraged to rate his wellbeing and lifestyle in the ten areas listed below, on a five-point scale. A score of *one* indicates very low wellbeing in an area, and a score of *five* indicates very high health status in this area.

- Emotional wellbeing
- Cognitive wellbeing
- Physical wellbeing
- Nutritional wellbeing
- Substance use wellbeing
- Sleep wellbeing
- Social/relationship wellbeing
- Spiritual wellbeing
- Illness self-management
- Readiness for change

Emotional wellbeing: Andre said that he was happy in his work and his marriage was solid, but worries about his health often lowered his mood and increased his anxiety. He rated himself a *two*.

Cognitive wellbeing: Andre rated himself as a *four* to *five*. He was proud of his college diploma and was functioning very well in a demanding job.

Physical wellbeing: Andre admitted that he was not as active as he should be and did not find the time for regular physical activity. He rated himself a *two* to *three*.

Nutritional wellbeing: Andre's food choices had improved since his physician suggested cutting down on salt and high-fat foods. But Andre was only eating two to three fruits or vegetables a day instead of the recommended five. He rated himself a *two* to *three*.

Substance use wellbeing: Andre drank moderately and did not use illegal drugs. He rated himself a *five*.

Sleep wellbeing: Andre had a solid sleep history until his diagnosis of hypertension. Recently, it took him more than an hour to fall asleep and he woke up several times during the night. His self-rating of sleep was *two*.

Social/relationship wellbeing: Andre had a solid marriage, good friends, and got along well with his co-workers and the staff who reported to him. He rated himself a *four* to *five*.

Spiritual wellbeing: Andre first hesitated, then asked what relevance his spirituality was to his blood pressure. The provider explained that spiritual wellbeing is not just defined as church attendance, but research supports positive effects of connection with the larger universe as being beneficial to health. Andre demurred at self-rating.

Illness self-management: Andre said he had tried to change his eating habits with some success, but his BP had not been lowered by changes in nutrition alone. The interviewer mentioned that self-management also included taking medication as prescribed and other lifestyle changes. Andre responded that he did take his medication but believed that he had little control over his cardiovascular health. He rated himself a *three*.

Readiness for change: Andre said he wanted to change his trajectory of worsening health and he hoped that Pathways could help him, but he admitted that he thought the chances of Pathways producing a significant change with long-term benefits were small. Nevertheless, he was willing to try. He rated himself a *two*.

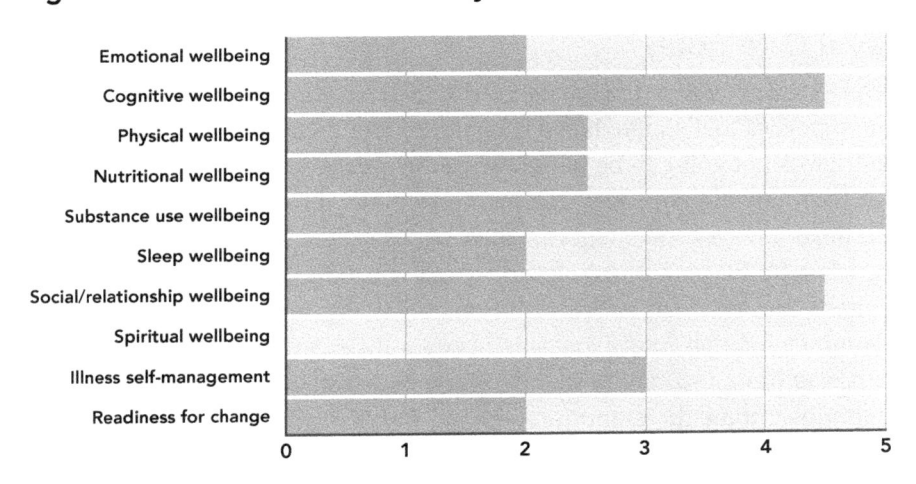

Figure 5.1: Andre's initial Pathways self-assessment

Category	Score
Emotional wellbeing	2
Cognitive wellbeing	4.5
Physical wellbeing	2.5
Nutritional wellbeing	2.5
Substance use wellbeing	5
Sleep wellbeing	2
Social/relationship wellbeing	4.5
Spiritual wellbeing	0
Illness self-management	3
Readiness for change	0

The Pathways team reviewed Andre's history from the medical record, his recent blood work, and the scores on the self-assessments. They saw the documentation of the last session with his physician where Andre had stated that he was "doomed". They contacted the physician and he gave the Pathways team further information. The physician remembered the conversation with Andre and expressed his concern that Andre might be suicidal, although he had denied it vehemently. The statements about "doom" were confusing to the physician when he knew there were so many available strategies to lower blood pressure.

The Pathways team was concerned about Andre's pervasive fatalism. They introduced Andre to the Healing Pathways Worksheet on "Heredity is Not Destiny". (The Healing Pathways Worksheets can be found in Appendix C.) Andre read the worksheet, filled it out with answers from his own life, and found it encouraging. He made a commitment to undertake some Pathways-based activities. Yet he also insisted that in the back of his mind, he still felt that God might just "call his number" and erase any effects of his healthy behaviors.

Pathways treatment
Level One goals
Level One involves setting goals for self-directed changes, including self-care practices and simple lifestyle changes. The Pathways team sensed that Andre was not going to be patient with the change process, so whatever was recommended in Level One had to give him a sense of empowerment and must have a good chance of success. The Level One interventions chosen were BP monitoring, lowering salt consumption, increasing aerobic exercise, and slow-paced breathing exercises. The behavioral specialist recommended that Andre measure his own BP at home, twice in each arm, with readings a few minutes apart, while in a seated position. Hopeful, Andre took home the monitoring device. To his dismay, however, the home pressures were equal or higher than those documented in the clinic. He refused to continue to do home measurements.

Level One goal: breathing
Slow, paced breathing was introduced with the rationale of gaining control over the breathing rate, which is known to also reduce BP. Andre began to practice slow breathing several times a day and reported that he felt calmer at work and particularly on audits when he had to give a corporate manager bad news.

Wellness program in the workplace
Andre remarked that his company was beginning a program to enhance the personal wellbeing of the accountants and staff. As a supervisor, his responsibility was to support the program – he was encouraged to participate and show leadership for his own staff. Andre questioned his boss about whether he needed to participate. His boss explained that the wellness program could not be made mandatory, but the program was important. Success would affect the company's insurance rates and would therefore save money.

Level One goal: salt reduction
The company wellness coach suggested a simple goal to begin the program: reduce salt. Information was provided about the salt content of common foods and the recommended amount of salt consumption per day (under 2,300 mg). Andre and his co-workers were shocked to discover that many seemingly "healthy" soups available from the vending machines contained 600-700mg of salt – and that was without the crackers that came with them.

The group took salt reduction as a challenge; they reported success and expressed pride in their new awareness. Changes were made to the contents of company vending machines. Andre bought this information home to Winnie, and she agreed to gradually reduce the amount of salt that she used in cooking. Andre allowed his BP to be measured by the wellness coach, and to his surprise, his BP had decreased a few points.

Level One goal: physical activity

The recommendation to increase physical activity was put on hold because Andre and his team left town on a three-week trip to conduct audits. On his return to the Pathways team, Andre expressed impatience with the program – he had an appointment scheduled with his physician and was sure that the doctor would pressure him to accept an increase in antihypertensive medication and the referral to cardiology. The team considered Andre's concerns and told him that he could move to Level Two, however he would need to commit more time and energy to the program. After a week of thought, Andre made that commitment.

Level Two goals

Level Two in the Pathways Program involves acquiring new coping skills and drawing on educational materials and community resources. Andre's Level Two goals were to increase his physical activity, improve nutrition, and minimize the effects of stress on his blood pressure. The specific interventions included mindfulness, additional relaxation practice, the DASH diet, and aerobic and strengthening exercises.

Level Two goal: nutrition

A dietician provided guidance for the Level Two nutritional goals. Winnie was brought into the initial session with the dietician, since she did most of the cooking for the family. Winnie and Andre had already reduced the salty snacks at home, but more changes were needed. Winnie was an enthusiastic learner; she had retained about twenty pounds after her pregnancies and wished to get back to her normal weight.

The dietician provided information about saturated fats and high-sugar beverages and recommended increasing fruits and vegetables to five portions per day. Andre commented that his grandmother and mother served cooked vegetables, but they were often mushy and had little flavour. Winnie always had raw carrots and celery for the kids' lunches but had not incorporated many cooked vegetables into the family's diet. Fresh fruit was viewed as expensive and often wasted, since it ripened before the family used it. Several shopping trips with the dietician were very helpful in planning meals and reducing waste. Sample meal plans and recipes were provided, and the dietician checked on progress with both Andre and Winnie on a weekly basis.

Level Two goal: stress management and heart rate variability training

Andre asked for additional help with stress management. The behavioral specialist noticed that Andre had a smart phone and commented that this could assist him in learning a powerful new tool for stress management: heart rate variability biofeedback. Heart rate variability (HRV) biofeedback is closely related to cardiovascular health; healthy hearts have greater variability in heart rate. A series of research studies have shown that when the variability of heart rate is low, patients with heart problems are more likely to suffer a heart attack and more likely to die. On the other hand, patients with higher variability are less likely to suffer a heart attack and will live longer. HRV is closely related to breathing, and a specialized form of breath training can increase HRV and increase heart health.

Andre's behavioral specialist guided him to download a breath pacer to his phone, and helped him set it at six breaths per minute. On average, this is the breathing rate that will best increase HRV. Andre now adapted his slow-breathing exercises to breathing with the pacer for two weeks, until he could breathe at this rate on demand, without the pacer. Then she loaned him a special HRV sensor, called Inner Balance™, from the Heart Math company. She helped him download the Inner Balance software to his phone, and then showed him how to continue his breathing and observe the effects of his breathing on his heart rate on the Inner Balance display. After two weeks with the Inner Balance, he was able to produce smooth large oscillations in his heart rate, visible on his phone. Andre was fascinated by the technology and by his increasing ability to change his own heart rhythms. He practiced his HRV exercises during times of relaxation but also during stressful times. He practiced daily and noticed significant improvement in his ability to increase his HRV. He reported falling asleep within thirty minutes and awakening in the morning feeling much more rested.

Level Two goal: mindfulness

Mindfulness training encourages total immersion in the moment without judgment. Mindfulness training was introduced as a way to help Andre reduce distracting thoughts about his health and focus on the moment. He had no trouble concentrating at work, but often ruminated about his risk factors for stroke and heart attack in the evenings after the kids went to bed. Andre used a mindfulness training CD developed by Jon Kabat-Zinn to practice formal mindfulness meditation and also to cultivate mindful acceptance in everyday life. He began to apply mindful acceptance during meals with the family. He noticed that meals with his family were more enjoyable if he was in the moment and not distracted by thoughts that he might not be at the table for much longer, because his death could come before the next meal. His focus on the food and comments about taste and texture of the newly introduced foods increased Winnie's motivation to continue to plan and cook healthier dinners.

Level Two goal: physical activity

Andre questioned the rationale for physical activity since exercise is well known to produce significant increases in blood pressure. Of course, Andre knew the research on the benefits of exercise and could quote the amount of reduction in BP that could be expected (5-7 mm Hg minimum), but his fear of any increase in blood pressure overruled his rational mind. The exercise physiologist knew Andre's history and carefully explained that blood pressure must increase during exercise to provide additional blood flow to the working muscles, and small blood vessels must dilate to accommodate an increase in blood flow. Regular exercise shortens recovery time after exercise and, over time, lowers resting blood pressure and reduces plaque formation in the arteries. Andre was satisfied with this explanation. At this same time, the wellness coach at Andre's office shifted the emphasis of the program to physical activity and recommended that, on rainy days, the accountants could use the onsite gym. Pick-up basketball games were fun, and within two months, there was a "league" and competitive games. Andre was not alone in the gym!

Level Two goal: nature engagement

The Pathways team considered the role of nature experiences in Andre's plan. It was spring and Andre was encouraged to spend more time outside enjoying the early signs and smells of new grass and budding flowers. He responded that he did not have time for this activity since he was physically active now – besides, he did not see how nature experiences could possibly help his blood pressure.

Level Three goals

Andre was praised for his success in Level Two. His BP had decreased to 130/85 mmHg. As Andre and the Pathways team considered Level Three interventions, they concluded that he would benefit from two professional interventions: a) continued consultation with his physician about antihypertensive medication, and b) a spiritual guide to directly address his conviction that nothing he could do would make a difference, because God would simply decide to take him as that long-ago sermon had suggested.

Level Three goal: medication

Andre's physician was encouraged by his lifestyle changes and the reductions in his blood pressure. He agreed to continue Andre on a single medication, unless his BP began to increase again.

Level Three goal: pastoral counseling

Andre was nervous about being judged by a minister, and considered seeing a psychotherapist affiliated with the Pathways team. However, the clinical psychologist felt that, although he might help Andre understand and manage his angry feelings, he did not feel qualified to act as a spiritual director, nor to help Andre with his sense of being doomed by God's decisions. There were several spiritual advisers on the referral list for Pathways; one was a young minister at a local Methodist church. Andre could also contact a trusted person at his own church. He refused this suggestion but agreed to meet with the young minister located close to the hospital complex.

Progress in Level Three

Andre returned for a follow-up appointment approximately two months after his last contact with the Pathways team. He brought a sense of calm into the room. He said he wanted to tell the team the complete story of the deaths in his family and his growing terror as he approached the age of fifty. He told of his unshakeable belief that God had vengeance in mind when He took this father and his grandfather.

He said the minister was kind and understanding; he did not confront Andre's beliefs. Instead, the minister provided education about the Old and New Testaments of the Bible. He explained that, in the Old Testament, there are many stories of violence and destruction, and God seems to be demanding retribution and even wanting people to suffer. The New Testament introduces the loving God. He encourages people to be active on their own behalf, to work, to have families, and to be happy. This God is compassionate and forgives sins. This God gave us nature; yet sometimes it seems that nature is angry and creates storms that hurt people and destroy property. However, when bad things happen to good people, God has not singled out the person to make them suffer. The minister recommended the book *When Bad Things Happen to Good People*, by Rabbi Harold Kushner, and Andre read it over and over.

The conversation about nature reminded Andre of the Pathways team's recommendation of nature experiences and his rejection of the suggestion. The minister said that connection with nature, and an appreciation of it, can be part of a spiritual journey, and often brings people closer to God. In addition, nature has been shown to help people improve mood, decrease anxiety, and improve physical health. Andre decided to add walks in local parks and natural areas to his Pathways self-care plans.

> *"The minister said that connection with nature, and appreciation of it, can be part of a spiritual journey and often brings people closer to God. In addition, nature has been shown to help people improve mood, decrease anxiety, and improve physical health."*

During their meetings, Andre recalled every detail of his father's funeral and he and the minister dissected every word. The minister interpreted the long-ago sermon as a way to explain the early death of a husband, father, and beloved community member. As a child, Andre only heard that God TOOK his father. He said:

> "I now believe that I do have control over my physiological and emotional reactions. My father was overweight and did not exercise. My grandfather smoked and drank too much. I can make (and have made) different choices and I will do everything I can to keep myself healthy. I enjoy my exercise, whether riding bikes with Andrell or playing basketball in the gym. When I spend time outdoors, I feel peaceful and closer to God. My prayer life is now much different; instead of always asking God why and feeling angry, now I pray for wisdom so that I can make good decisions about my health. My recent appointment with my doctor was encouraging. I have

lost fifteen pounds, and my blood pressure at that checkup was 120/80 mmHg. He did not increase my medication. I continue to use mindfulness meditation (formal and informal), and my phone apps for relaxation. I accepted the referral to a cardiologist to find out what else I can do to prevent heart disease and stroke.

"I believe that God has a plan, but my decisions are part of that plan. My heredity for heart disease is strong on my father's side; but strangely enough, I never considered my mother's side. She is still alive, and my grandmother lived into her seventies. My mother has arthritis and sometimes it flares up, but there is no history of cardiovascular disease on her side. Why did I never consider that aspect of my heredity? I was overwhelmed with fear and the fear clouded my rational mind. Ironic, since I use my mathematical, logical mind in my work. Thank you for your patience with me. And thank you for suggesting that a major problem was a spiritual crisis that needed a spiritual guide to help me resolve it.

"I sat down with Andrell last week and had an honest open conversation with him about his heredity on both sides of the family. I emphasized personal control and good decision making. He took it very well and did not show any fear. I have broken the chain of fear and hopelessness in my family."

Level Three interventions involve professional medical, psychiatric, psychological, pastoral counseling, or other services and treatments. Andre benefitted from two Level Three interventions: antihypertensive medication, and his meetings with the spiritual adviser.

Final Pathways assessment

Andre agreed to rate himself again on each of the ten areas in his initial assessment, to see more clearly his progress in lifestyle and wellbeing, and to recognize any areas that might need continued attention.

Emotional wellbeing: Andre said that he was much calmer and that he was no longer tortured by memories of the past. The overwhelming anxiety that he had experienced when he had his blood pressure measured or when he thought of his future was gone. He still worried about his health, but the thoughts did not overwhelm him. He rated himself a *four*.

Cognitive wellbeing: Andre again rated himself as a *four* to *five*. He continued to be very productive at his work.

Physical wellbeing: Andre was pleased with his physical activity. He rode bikes with his son, played basketball in the gym at work, and had increased his use of weights for strengthening his muscles. He rated himself as a *five* in physical activity.

Nutritional wellbeing: Andre's choices of foods were much healthier and his consumption of high-fat, high-sugar, and high-salt foods had decreased significantly. He rated himself a *four* and then laughingly said that Winnie was a *five* because she had lost twenty pounds!

Substance use wellbeing: There was no change in his normal use of alcohol. He rated himself a *five*.

Sleep wellbeing: Andre's sleep had improved. He could fall asleep easily after using his breathing exercise. He rarely woke up except to use the bathroom and arose feeling rested. He was sleep deprived during his travel weeks but was able to restore normal sleep after returning home. He rated himself a *four*.

Social/relationship wellbeing: Andre had a solid marriage, friends, and got along well with his co-workers and the staff who reported to him. He rated himself a *four* to *five*.

Spiritual wellbeing: Andre was more at peace and had returned to church with his family. When the thoughts of doom came into his mind, he now prayed for a long and healthy life. He knew he would need to continue to work on deepening his faith. He rated himself a *three* to *four*.

Illness self-management: Andre was taking his antihypertensive medication and followed his nutritional and activity plan. His BP had decreased to 120/80 mm Hg in the provider's office and at home. He rated himself a *four*.

Readiness for change: Andre stated his commitment to maintain his newly earned normal blood pressure. He accepted the fact that blood pressure may increase again, but he would follow his physician's recommendations and continue his lifestyle modifications. He rated himself a *four*.

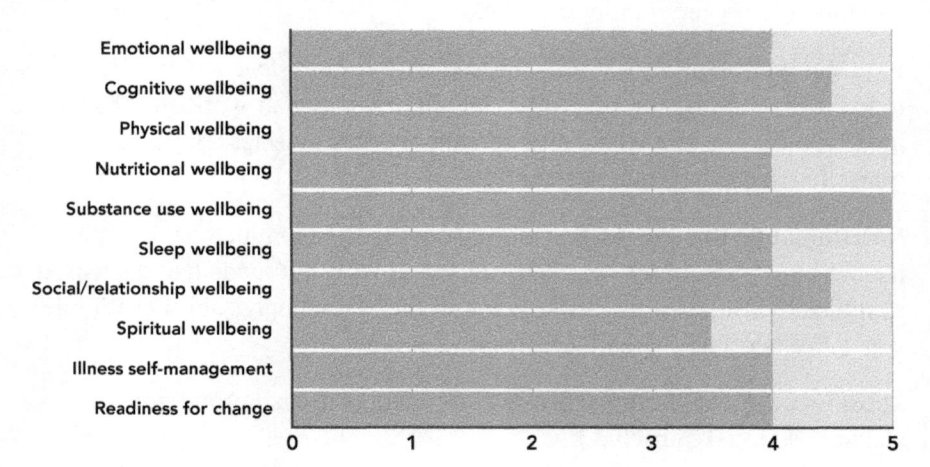

Figure 5.2: Andre's final Pathways self-assessment

Emotional wellbeing	
Cognitive wellbeing	
Physical wellbeing	
Nutritional wellbeing	
Substance use wellbeing	
Sleep wellbeing	
Social/relationship wellbeing	
Spiritual wellbeing	
Illness self-management	
Readiness for change	

Conclusion

Knowledge of heredity gives a person more control, since decisions about exercise, food choices, stress management, and the use of substances can be made based on reliable data. With very few exceptions, genetics is not destiny. In any disorder in which stress or other aspects of lifestyle influence the development, trajectory, or response to treatment of illness, the person can moderate the severity of the health condition and reduce the risk of early death. However, what a child hears and misinterprets about the causes of death during a time of intense sadness affects adult behavior. This chapter used hypertension as an example of an inheritable chronic illness strongly influenced by lifestyle. The Pathways Model offers a comprehensive approach to the management of high blood pressure. It addresses family history, traumatic memories, and current lifestyle. Negative lifestyle effects can be changed through education, intention to change, reasonable goals, and behavior modification. Yet, Andre's motivation resembled a ticking clock, with his perceived threats of worsening hypertension, developing heart disease, and a belief that death could come at any time.

The benefits of the interventions in Levels One and Two were significant, but progress stopped because of Andre's unshakeable belief that God's plan and heredity were the main factors determining his life span. Referral to a spiritual adviser was the best choice for Andre as his primary

Pathways Level Three intervention. He needed someone with extensive knowledge of the Bible and spiritual practices who could re-interpret his memories of the sermon at his father's funeral. The minister was known to the Pathways team. He supported many of Andre's Level One and Level Two interventions, but also provided the very important spiritual guidance that Andre needed. As his sense of doom diminished, Andre also cooperated more easily with his physician's medication management and with a referral to a cardiologist, to better understand his heart disease risk.

Final message: *Heredity is important, yet heredity is not destiny. The Pathways Model guides patients to adopt self-care practices and lifestyle changes that can moderate the severity of chronic illness and prolong life. Pathways-based behavioral changes can reduce distress and greatly enhance one's quality of life. At the same time, implementing medical advice and accepting medication targeting one's illness is important in managing any chronic condition. Andre also needed pastoral counseling to overcome his fears of a punishing God and to regain hope both in God and in his own ability to manage his condition. Spiritual interventions can be a critical tool for effective integrative healthcare.*

Resources

Frates, B., Tollefson, M., & Comander, A. (2021). *Paving the Path to Wellness Workbook*. Healthy Learning.

Kabat-Zinn, J. (2002a). *Guided Mindfulness Meditation* (series 1). (Audio CD). Better Listening LLC.

Kabat-Zinn, J. (2002b). *Guided Mindfulness Meditation* (series 2). (Audio CD). Better Listening LLC.

Kabat-Zinn, J. (1994). *Wherever You Go, There You Are: Mindfulness meditation in everyday life*. Hyperion.

Kushner, H. S. (2004). *When Bad Things Happen to Good People* (reprint edition). Anchor Books.

Potter-Efron, R. (2012). *Healing the angry brain*. New Harbinger Publications.

Unger, T. Borghi, C., Charchar, F., et al. (2020). International Society of Hypertension global hypertension practice guidelines. *Journal of Hypertension*, **38**(6), 984-1004.

Vemu, P. L., Yang, E., Ebinger, J. (2024, February). 2023 ESH hypertension guideline update: Bringing us closer together across the pond. American College of Cardiology. Available at: www.acc.org/Latest-in-Cardiology/Articles/2024/02/05/11/43/2023-ESH-Hypertension-Guideline-Update#:~:text=The%202023%20ESH%20guidelines%20maintain,the%202018%20ESC%2FESH%20guidelines.&text=The%20ESH%20recommends%20a%20threshold,mm%20Hg%20(stage%201) (accessed September 2024).

Williams, F. (2018). *The Nature Fix*. W. W. Norton.

Useful websites

American College of Lifestyle Medicine. https://lifestylemedicine.org

American Heart Association. www.heart.org

American Heart Association. (2023). Managing blood pressure with a heart-healthy diet. Health Topics. Available at: www.heart.org/en/health-topics/high-blood-pressure/changes-you-can-make-to-manage-high-blood-pressure/managing-blood-pressure-with-a-heart-healthy-diet (accessed September 2024)

American Heart Association. (2024). High blood pressure. Health Topics. Available at: www.heart.org/en/health-topics/high-blood-pressure (accessed September 2024).

Cleveland Clinic (2022). How exercise helps lower blood pressure and eight activities to try. Health Essentials. https://health.clevelandclinic.org/exercises-to-lower-blood-pressure (accesed September 2024).

Cleveland Clinic (2022). Six types of foods that lower blood pressure. Health Essentials. Available at: https://health.clevelandclinic.org/foods-to-lower-blood-pressure (accessed September 2024).

Levi, A. (2023). What is the DASH diet? Health Newsletters. Available at: www.health.com/dash-diet-7972360 (accessed September 2024).

Mayo Clinic Staff. (2024). DASH diet: Healthy eating to lower your blood pressure. Nutrition and Healthy Eating. Mayo Clinic. Available at: www.mayoclinic.org/healthy-lifestyle/nutrition-and-healthy-eating/in-depth/dash-diet/art-20048456 (accessed September 2024).

National Institutes of Health. (no date). DASH eating plan. Available at: www.nhlbi.nih.gov/education/dash-eating-plan (accessed September 2024).

Chapter 6:
Embracing nature and recovering inner peace (cancer)

Summary: Living with a long-term condition frequently brings an end to once-positive activities such as walking in a park, visiting the beach, hiking, bicycling, and other physical pastimes. This chapter uses cancer as an example to illustrate how illness can undermine a person's quality of life, and to show pathways to recover joy and fulfilment in a life with illness.

Cancer is a family of disorders, categorized by the organs in the body affected by cancer, and also by the type of cancer cell involved. Cancer continues to be a frightening word for most people, yet with early identification and more effective treatments, the death rates for many cancers are declining and average survival times are increasing.

The chapter introduces the case of Maddie, a sixty-six-year-old retired schoolteacher, and illustrates the application of the Pathways Model to uterine cancer. Maddie used a variety of self-care techniques and lifestyle choices to manage the effects of chemotherapy and radiation, regain control of her life, and live as fully as possible with her illness.

Keywords: cancer, Pathways Model, nature, lifestyle, spirituality, heart rate variability, paced breathing

Healing theme: embracing nature and recovering inner peace

Living with a long-term condition frequently brings an end to once-positive activities such as walking in a park, visiting the beach, bicycling, and other physical pastimes. Immersion in nature and vigorous physical activities are sources of joy and renewal for many healthy people, and their loss lowers their quality of life. Instead, many people with long-term illness describe their social life as keeping medical appointments, visiting physical therapy, and submitting to lab tests. Others with long-term conditions, however, do retain some immersion in nature and at least a moderately active lifestyle.

> *"Living with a long-term condition frequently brings an end to once-positive activities such as walking in a park, visiting the beach, bicycling, and other physical pastimes."*

This chapter uses cancer as an example to illustrate both how illness can undermine quality of life, and to show pathways to recover joy and fulfilment within a life with illness. Cancer is a family of disorders, categorized by the organs in the body affected by cancer, and by the type of cancer cell involved. Cancer continues to be a frightening word for most people, yet, with early identification and more effective treatments, the death rates for many cancers are declining and average survival times are increasing. Today, the challenge for individuals with a cancer diagnosis is to work collaboratively with a team of health professionals and manage the effects of the illness as well as the adverse effects of cancer treatments.

Understanding cancer

Cancer can be defined as an illness in which the body develops abnormal cells which divide and increase in the body. These cancer cells become a danger to the body as they invade and damage healthy tissues. Medical doctors categorize cancers according to *anatomical site and histology*, that is, in what organ the cancer develops, and what kind of cancer cells are involved. So, we diagnose breast cancer, lung cancer, prostate cancer, stomach cancer, pancreatic cancer, and other varieties, because the cancer occurs in these organs. Cancers are then rated by the size of the tumour, whether the cancer has spread outside the original organ, and whether the cancer cells have *metastasized* to other, perhaps distant, parts of the body. We also use laboratory analysis to study the cancer cells and categorize them by type. A cancer in the breast can be caused by several types of cells. The size of the tumour, the degree to which it is contained, the presence of distant metastases, and the histology or cell type all affect the prognosis, the prediction of recovery, and the likely survival time.

For the patient with a new cancer diagnosis, it is useful to learn about cancer, but important not to be overly concerned about cancer statistics. Prognosis has to do with group averages and does not always determine your personal fate. There are long-term survivors and individuals who continue to live very fully, in every category of cancer illness. It is important for the patient to learn about self-care practices, coping skills, and lifestyle factors that can counteract the adverse effects of cancer treatments, mobilize the body's immune system for longer-term survival, and improve the quality of life.

> *"Today, the challenge for the individual with a cancer diagnosis is to work collaboratively with a team of health professionals and manage the effects of the illness as well as the adverse effects of cancer treatments."*

In 2020, according to the National Cancer Institute, approximately 1.8 million people were diagnosed with cancer in the USA alone, and approximately 600,000 died from it. The most common cancers are breast cancer, lung and bronchial cancer, prostate cancer, colon and rectal cancer, melanoma of the skin, bladder cancer, non-Hodgkin lymphoma, kidney and renal pelvic cancer, endometrial cancer, leukaemia, pancreatic cancer, thyroid cancer, and liver cancer. The incidence of cancer is similar for men and women, but men are more likely to die of cancer. About 39% of men and women will likely face a cancer diagnosis at some time in their lives. Prostate, lung, and colorectal cancers account for about 43% of the cancers in men, and breast, lung, and colorectal cancers account for more than 50% of cancers in women.

Survival times for men and women are increasing, due both to earlier diagnosis and more effective treatments. The cost of cancer care is increasing dramatically, both because individuals with cancer are living longer, and because new cancer medications and surgical techniques come with higher price tags. However, a variety of inexpensive self-directed self-care practices, coping skills, and lifestyle choices can greatly enhance quality of life and contribute to managing the illness.

Introducing Maddie

Maddie was a vibrant and athletic sixty-six-year-old when she was diagnosed with cancer. She retired from elementary school teaching but was actively involved with her husband's family business, a marina crowded with power boats and sailboats. She was an avid camper and hiker and had visited and hiked in many national parks. An episode of breakthrough bleeding led Maddie to see her gynaecologist, and a pelvic exam led to an endometrial ultrasound, and then an immediate referral to a gynaecological oncologist. At each stage, more concerns were raised until a hysterectomy and biopsy of a large tumour showed a carcinosarcoma of the uterus, a high-risk cancer not entirely contained in the uterus. The uterus and ovaries were completely removed in the surgery. Her oncologist recommended intensive in-hospital chemotherapy to be followed by several months of outpatient radiation and outpatient chemotherapy.

Maddie saw a "nurse navigator" at the cancer centre before surgery, a nurse specially trained to help the cancer patient understand the illness and find her way through the confusing maze of clinics, hospitals, and healthcare providers. Her nurse navigator was familiar with the Pathways Model and suggested that Maddie begin some discussions of self-care and lifestyle options, while in the hospital for surgery. Betty, the nurse navigator, had experience guiding cancer patients through times of anxiety, reactions to chemotherapy, and other cancer-related challenges.

The Pathways journey: assessment

The first step for Maddie, while in the hospital recovering from surgery, was a Pathways Assessment, assisted by her nurse navigator. The assessment includes documenting strengths and weaknesses in several areas listed below:

- Emotional wellbeing
- Cognitive wellbeing
- Physical wellbeing
- Nutritional wellbeing
- Substance use wellbeing
- Sleep wellbeing
- Social/relationship wellbeing
- Spiritual wellbeing
- Illness self-management
- Readiness for change

Maddie's assessment was different from that of most patients with long-term illnesses, as the typical person with chronic illness experiences many years of declining activity and increasing impact of illness. Maddie was suddenly informed of a new condition, cancer, which threatened to become a lingering presence impacting her life. Yet she had been living a full, active lifestyle until the day of hospitalization.

Emotional wellbeing: Maddie decided she was suffering from *emotional whiplash*. She didn't feel depressed or particularly anxious. But she felt in shock and a bit confused at how her life had taken a sudden left turn, without any warning. Her calendar told her she should be in Glacier National Park hiking and viewing bear habitat, but she was instead in hospital recovering from surgery and discussing a major project of lifestyle change and recovery. She rated her emotional wellbeing as a *three* on a one-to-five-point scale (with one indicating disabling negative emotions and five indicating high emotional wellness). She decided to simply continue to monitor her emotional state, realizing she might feel more distress later.

Cognitive wellbeing: At the time of assessment, Maddie's cognitive state was sharp and alert, with good focus. She rated herself as a *five*, indicating high mental wellness. She remained concerned about her thinking because she understood that chemotherapy often produces loss of alertness, cognitive deficits, and "brain fog".

Physical wellbeing: Maddie had been highly active before her cancer diagnosis but then quickly reduced her activity. In her mind, she saw herself as fragile and vulnerable. She rated herself as a *two* on physical activity, indicating a new low level of physical wellbeing. Her goal was to recover her confidence in her body and resume activity during recovery. Yet she was fearful of her body's response to the cancer treatments and felt grief for her once athletic lifestyle.

Nutritional wellbeing: Maddie characterized her nutrition as lazy and unhealthy. She rated herself as a *one* in nutrition, indicating a severely unhealthy diet. Because she was spending many hours at the family marina, she had developed habits of eating most breakfasts and lunches out and dining on take-out meals most evenings. Maddie was slightly underweight for her height, but she and her husband had frequently discussed improving their nutrition for their health. They never acted on the idea.

Substance use wellbeing: Maddie often worked twelve-hour shifts at the marina and regularly drank twelve or more servings of cola and coffee daily. The caffeine helped her stay alert working the cash register and doing bookkeeping but left her jittery and contributed to poor sleep onset and fragmented sleep. She drank only an occasional glass of wine and used no tobacco, recreational drugs, or habit-forming prescription medications. She rated herself as a *three* in overall substance use, because she did not use drugs, used alcohol moderately, but abused caffeine daily.

Sleep wellbeing: Maddie had a long history of delayed sleep onset and restless, fragmented sleep, even before her caffeine use increased. She slept much better on vacations, usually camping and hiking, away from the business. She felt adequately rested to function most mornings, but her afternoon caffeine use had increased greatly in recent years. She rated herself as a *two*, indicating poor sleep, with several years of sleep disturbance.

Social/relationship wellbeing: Maddie was close to her brother, three sisters, and three grown children, but they all lived where the family had grown up, while Maddie had moved in her fifties with her current husband. She had several close girlfriends from her last teaching job, and they continued to see one another frequently in retirement. Her marina work hours had increased after a recent expansion, and she now found it harder to meet friends or have much of a couples' social life. She trusted that her friends would be there for her if she needed help during treatment. She rated herself as a *three* in social and relationship wellbeing, based on her infrequent contact with friends in recent years.

Spiritual wellbeing: Maddie grew up with a strict, sin and judgment-oriented church and attended Sunday school, but she drifted away from any religious life over her adult years. She reported that she was suddenly praying again and trying to talk to God about her medical problems. First, she prayed that she would not have cancer, and now was praying for the strength to cope with the illness and treatments. She wished for some kind of more positive spiritual help as part of her self-care but was apprehensive that any renewed religious activity would lead to being condemned as a sinner again, as in childhood. She rated herself as a *two* in spiritual wellbeing, because she rarely engaged in spiritual practices, and had dropped formal religious activity in her adult years.

> *"She wished for some kind of more positive spiritual help as part of her self-care but was apprehensive that any renewed religious activity would lead to being condemned as a sinner again, as in childhood."*

Self-management and readiness for change: Maddie saw herself as a decisive person who was used to stepping into problem situations and taking charge. She felt that her illness was a wake-up call, and she felt ready to set some new goals and act on them. She committed to meeting with her nurse navigator weekly as an assurance of her commitment to serious changes in her life. She rated herself as a *five* on both illness self-management and readiness for change. She had always cooperated fully with medical care and felt ready and fully engaged with her nurse navigator and the initial discussions of self-care and lifestyle change.

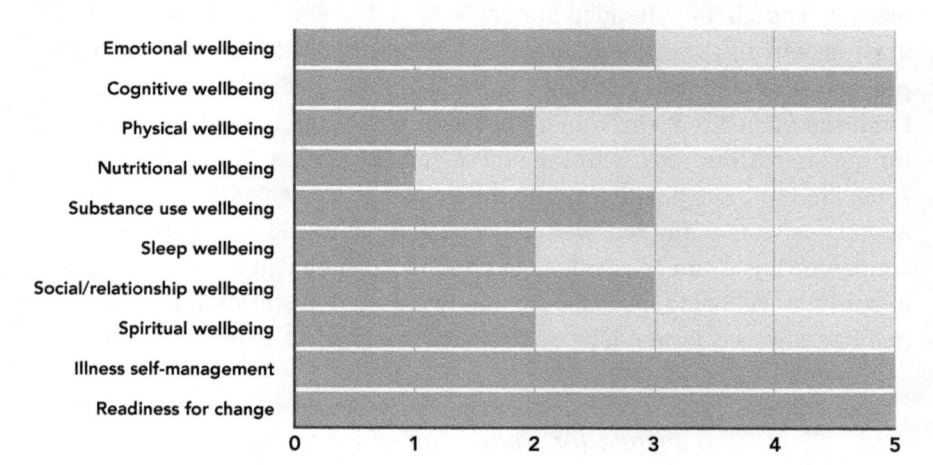

Figure 6.1: Maddie's initial Pathways self-assessment

Category	Score
Emotional wellbeing	3
Cognitive wellbeing	5
Physical wellbeing	2
Nutritional wellbeing	1
Substance use wellbeing	5
Sleep wellbeing	2
Social/relationship wellbeing	3
Spiritual wellbeing	2
Illness self-management	5
Readiness for change	3

Pathways treatment

Level One goals

Level One involves setting goals for self-directed changes, including self-care practices and simple lifestyle changes. Maddie decided to focus some of her Level One and Level Two goals on practices that would help her cope with chemotherapy and radiation.

Level One goal: breathing

Betty, the nurse navigator, explained to Maddie that in-hospital platinum-based chemotherapy, which she would undergo, is one of the harshest forms of chemotherapy, fighting cancer cells aggressively, but stressful for the body and the mind. Platinum-based agents typically trigger nausea, raise blood pressure, disrupt kidney function, produce cognitive deficits, and induce a range of other side effects. Betty taught Maddie paced diaphragmatic breathing, as a tool to diminish nausea and relax through the cancer treatment process. Cancer care is stressful, and stress reduction is beneficial for keeping the immune system functioning at its best.

Level One goal: guided imagery

Ordinarily, the use of educational CDs, downloads, and other resources are Level Two interventions. However, because Maddie was facing in-hospital chemotherapy within two weeks, Betty loaned her several educational CDs from Bellaruth Naparstek, a social worker who specializes in guided imagery. Naparstek has produced useful CDs and other materials for coping with cancer, reducing chemotherapy-related nausea, and general relaxation. Maddie committed to listening to three CDs in rotation, listening for twenty minutes at least twice daily, commencing immediately. Betty suggested that while in the hospital for chemotherapy, Maddie listened to the CDs in every unscheduled moment.

Level One goal: nutrition

Maddie wanted to focus a Level One goal on improving her unhealthy nutrition. She took an indefinite leave from work at the marina to accommodate her treatments and realized she would be recovering at home for much of the next few weeks. So, making changes in nutrition seemed more possible at this time. Maddie ended up with two nutritional goals. She decided to reduce her caffeine intake, only having coffee with breakfast. She would not need caffeine to focus if she were not working. Maddie also decided to prepare more meals at home herself, to make her nutrition healthier. She had read online that just preparing one's own meals can produce a significant health effect.

Level One progress

Maddie made progress initially, learning to self-calm via paced slow breathing and practicing guided imagery daily. She liked the Naparstek CDs and the imagery they contained. She felt more confident facing the chemotherapy. She purchased some grains and fresh vegetables and began gathering recipes for healthy home-cooked meals.

During her initial hospitalization, the chemotherapy affected Maddie far more than she expected. She found herself unable to focus, unable to guide herself in paced breathing, and unable to listen to the imagery CDs. Her blood pressure peaked several times during the hospitalization, at levels around 240/140. Her nausea was overwhelming, and it was challenging for her to do her self-care, even challenging to answer her physician's questions.

Betty, the nurse navigator, visited Maddie during an episode of extreme nausea. Initially, she guided Maddie in paced breathing, and then guided her, in her own voice, into a guided imagery relaxation exercise. Maddie's eyes were unfocused, and she apologized, saying "I can't".

> *"Maddie also decided to prepare more meals at home herself, to make her nutrition healthier. She had read online, that just preparing one's own meals can produce a significant health effect."*

Betty decided to try something new, brought her laptop out of her bag, attached a sensor to Maddie's index finger, and used a program in the laptop to guide Maddie. The program was called emWavePro®, from the HeartMath Institute. The computer showed Maddie a hot air balloon, and Betty asked Maddie to breathe slowly and make the balloon fly. Initially, Maddie continued crying, but after about five minutes, she saw the hot air balloon moving aloft and moving across the landscape. Maddie's breathing slowed and became more even, and the balloon moved higher and faster across the landscape. Maddie stayed with the computer program for about ten minutes and was more focused mentally by the end of the exercise. She also reported diminished nausea and a sense of moderate calm.

The emWavePro® program is a heart rate variability biofeedback training program. The sensor monitors moment-to-moment variations in heart rate, and slow-paced breathing serves to organize the heart rate variability (HRV), increasing the moment-to-moment oscillations in heart rate. Practice of this HRV training exercise helps many individuals counteract the effects of stress and produce better physiological regulation with many benefits for health and wellbeing. The presence of a computer display with animations, such as the hot air balloon ride, often helps individuals like Maddie, who for whatever reason cannot focus and self-regulate spontaneously.

Betty encouraged Maddie's spouse to download the HeartMath program on his own laptop, loaned him a HeartMath emWave Pro finger sensor, and helped him order a sensor for home use.[4] Maddie's spouse assisted her in doing the HRV training exercises several times a day in the hospital and guided her particularly to do the HeartMath exercises whenever the nausea increased. He and Maddie used the HeartMath exercises, the paced breathing, and the Naparstek imagery CDs through four inpatient chemotherapy regimens, and during the initial period of outpatient radiation.

---

[4] The HeartMath company also has an InnerBalance® device, a heart rate variability sensor that interacts with a smart phone or tablet. There are now many other heart rate variability devices and apps, available for purchase by the general public.

Level Two goals

Maddie was now in outpatient radiation. She saw the benefits from her paced slow breathing, guided imagery, and HeartMath HRV practices. She was happy with her initial efforts to reduce caffeine and improve her overall nutrition and was committed to continuing each of her Level One practices. However, she felt eager to go on to Pathways Level Two activities. Level Two goals continue to emphasize self-care but draw more extensively on external assistance and community-based resources.

Level Two goal: aquatherapy

Maddie experienced weakness in her legs and overwhelming fatigue during the weeks of her radiation therapy. Her oncologist recommended she remain active, walking and exercising moderately, yet she felt a complete loss of motivation for her previous activities. Her primary care physician referred her to a water-based exercise program, supervised by physical therapists, to maintain muscle strength and restore comfort with exercise. She signed up for a twice-weekly program of gentle exercise in a therapeutic pool.

Level Two goal: additional nutritional goals

Maddie was satisfied with herself for cooking more home-cooked dinners. She felt that she and her husband were eating much healthier than before her cancer diagnosis. However, she had looked online and found a confusing array of suggestions about specific foods and diets to enhance immune function and fight cancer. She wanted to do more nutritionally but was frustrated by the contradictory information.

Maddie's nurse navigator suggested she buy Rebecca Katz's book, *Cancer Fighting Kitchen*. This book presents basic concepts on how nutrition can enhance immune function and assist recovery from cancer. The book includes more than 150 recipes to stimulate appetite and moderate the adverse effects of cancer treatments. Maddie read the introduction to the book and decided to cook four to five Katz recipes each week as a Level Two goal. She also committed herself to further reducing caffeine intake to one to two cups of coffee a day.

Level Two goal: spiritual renewal

Cancer had triggered a new interest in spirituality for Maddie. She had no interest in returning to the hellfire and brimstone church of her girlhood, yet she wanted to pray and talk to God, and find a new sense of purpose in her life. Maddie made inquiries in her community and identified a retreat centre that offered spiritually oriented women's retreats. The retreat centre's brochure described learning meditation practices, using biblical imagery for emotional and physical healing, and spiritual conversations with the retreat participants, facilitated by one of the centre's spiritual guides. She signed up for a three-day retreat and determined that she could fit it into her radiation schedule.

Level Two goal: nature engagement

Maddie had been a "nature freak" (her term), boating, hiking, and exploring national parks. She estimated that she previously spent twenty nights a year sleeping under the stars. Since her cancer diagnosis, she suddenly saw herself as fragile and vulnerable and had cancelled all of her "roughing it". Maddie's nurse navigator gave her a Healing Pathways Worksheet to complete, to assess her engagement with nature. (See Appendix C for the Healing Pathways Worksheets.) She reviewed the worksheet and set an initial goal to take a walk at least once a week in the sand dunes at a beach near her home.

Level Two progress

Maddie was greatly encouraged by her participation in the water-based exercise program. The warm water relaxed her thoroughly as she exercised, and she found that the more she exercised in the pool, the more her energy returned. There were still days when she had no strength and could only exercise for a few minutes at a time, but these were now less frequent.

Maddie and her husband loved the Rebecca Katz recipes, with their emphasis on combining great nutrition and fabulous taste. She cooked twenty-four different Katz recipes in her first month and sipped on the Katz mineral broth as her new beverage of choice. She felt increased strength and energy with these healthier foods and was determined to continue more home cooking long term.

> *"Maddie was greatly encouraged by her participation in the water-based exercise program. The warm water relaxed her thoroughly as she exercised, and she found that the more she exercised in the pool, the more her energy returned."*

Maddie enjoyed the three-day women's retreat and signed up for a follow-up weekly meditation class. However, she quickly learned that many religious terms set off mini-panic attacks for her. Comments by other participants in the meditation class, about their church involvement, were highly disturbing for Maddie. She came to recognize how much her childhood religious training had left painful and traumatic memories. She decided for the time being to emphasize a meditation practice and encounters with nature as her primary spiritual practices. She experimented with praying but kept her prayers short, ending them whenever they triggered fear or upset. Maddie followed through almost every week on her goal of taking a walk in the nearby sand dunes. She found that this time in nature soothed her, moderated her physical tensions, and seemed to support a comfortable spiritual awareness, without the emotional pain that formal religious discussion triggered for her.

Level Three goals

Level Three involves selecting professional services and treatments to address one's long-term illness and any troublesome symptoms. Level Three treatments include mainstream medical care, complementary and integrative therapies, and spiritual support. Maddie selected three Level Three treatments: acupuncture, an energy-medicine-based therapy, and pastoral counseling.

Level Three treatment: acupuncture

Maddie's nausea moderated with her use of paced breathing, imagery, and heart rate variability exercises, but was not gone. She still experienced intense nausea each time she returned to the cancer centre for checkups or outpatient chemotherapy. Medical research has shown that acupuncture is moderately effective in reducing nausea before and following chemotherapy sessions. Maddie decided to use acupuncture as one of her Level Three treatments. She scheduled an initial visit with an osteopathic physician who was also trained in acupuncture.

> *"Level Three involves selecting professional services and treatments to address one's long-term illness and any troublesome symptoms. Level Three treatments include mainstream medical care, complementary and integrative therapies, and spiritual supports."*

Level Three treatment: energy therapy

Maddie was fascinated by the concept of *energy therapy* and *energy medicine*. She learned that a certified Reiki healer was available through the retreat centre. Reiki healers work with the human energy field, to change and balance the flow of energy in the person. Many cancer patients use Reiki healing to deal with the stress and tensions of cancer care and to optimize their wellbeing. Maddie was encouraged by several participants in her meditation class who had used Reiki. She signed up for weekly Reiki sessions for eight consecutive weeks.

Level Three treatment: pastoral counseling

Maddie was still upset that she had such negative emotions in reaction to many religious words and images. She scheduled an initial meeting with the minister who headed the retreat centre, and after the initial visit, agreed to several sessions of pastoral counseling to reduce her anxiety around religious memories and facilitate a less troubled relationship with God.

Progress in Level Three

The acupuncture practitioner recommended a series of sessions to include both acupuncture and acupressure. In acupuncture, the practitioner inserts fine needles along the energy meridians of the body, intending to facilitate energy flow, following principles of traditional Chinese medicine. After sessions of acupuncture, Maddie felt a reduction in nausea and a sense of calm. One day, she felt quite ill going into her session, like the onset of flu, and after acupuncture, she felt well again.

In acupressure, the practitioner uses manual pressure on meridian points to produce benefits. The acupuncturist showed Maddie and her husband how to apply manual pressure at the Neiguan point, a site on the inner arm near the wrist. Maddie's husband was more effective than Maddie at applying pressure, and whenever she experienced nausea at home, he applied pressure to the same site, and the nausea moderated.

Maddie was initially sceptical of her Reiki sessions. She could not feel anything happening and wondered if it was just a sham. After three sessions, she began to feel a kind of warmth and serenity whenever the Reiki therapist placed her hand on Maddie's torso and head.

The warmth permeated her musculature and soothed muscle stiffness and weakness. The Reiki therapy seemed to create the kind of serene mental state that Maddie was experiencing in meditation.

Maddie made progress in her pastoral counseling as well. She identified some key childhood memories of her minister screaming at her about hellfire and of the same minister insisting she watch as he whipped her brother with a belt for "backtalk". The retreat centre director was certified in EMDR, a therapeutic technique for resolving traumatic memories. EMDR stands for *eye movement desensitization and reprocessing* and involves the therapist guiding the client's eyes in side-to-side eye movements while the client remembers painful events. The technique worked rapidly for Maddie. After five sessions of EMDR and two additional sessions of talking through the memories, she found she could talk to God in prayer with no sense of shock or pain. Maddie scheduled a second retreat for herself, and this time engaged more extensively in dialogue with other participants, without stirring up any negative emotions.

Maddie's Pathways program assisted her in coping with the period of intensive cancer treatment. After Maddie completed both her outpatient radiation and outpatient chemotherapy, she was gradually able to recover more normality in her life. She and her husband took several day hikes around the area where they lived. She resumed walking and bicycling regularly and felt more like herself. She resumed bookkeeping at the family marina but made it clear that her working week was now 16 hours. After her cancer diagnosis, she wanted time free to enjoy living.

Maddie continued to practice paced breathing and guided imagery whenever she had a few free minutes. She developed a morning meditation practice and experimented with several new meditation techniques. She used the HeartMath emWave device intermittently, whenever she felt she was losing her effectiveness in self-guided relaxation.

Maddie experiences nausea less often now. Certain foods triggered nausea, as did return visits to the cancer centre. She was able to reliably manage the nausea by paced breathing and acupressure. She continued home cooking and felt able to enjoy eating in a way that was impossible during treatment.

> *"The healing themes in this chapter include incorporating nature, specifically walks in natural settings, the cycle of nature, rebirth each spring, and daylight. Maddie found that resuming her self-immersion in nature, especially taking walks in the nearby dunes, promoted her inner peace and energized her for self-care activities."*

Her spiritual practices were rewarding for Maddie for the first time in her life. She felt she was now in a time of spiritual searching, looking for a sense of purpose for the next phase in her life. The healing themes in this chapter include incorporating nature, specifically walks in natural settings, the cycle of nature, rebirth each spring, and daylight. Maddie found that resuming her self-immersion in nature, especially taking walks in the nearby dunes, promoted her inner peace and energized her for self-care activities.

Final Pathways assessment

Maddie completed a final Pathways self-assessment based on the same Pathways Assessment areas as in her initial self-assessment. She rated herself as follows:

Emotional wellbeing: She rated herself as a *four*, improved, and still working on it.

Cognitive wellbeing: She rated herself as a *five* on her cognition. She continued to think clearly and work efficiently.

Physical wellbeing: Maddie rated herself as a *five* on physical wellbeing, with her activity nearly fully recovered to pre-cancer levels.

Nutritional wellbeing: She rated herself as a *four* on nutrition. She had made much progress and continued to develop new coping strategies to manage nausea.

Substance use wellbeing: She rated herself as a *four-and-a-half* on substance use, with only occasional caffeine intake.

Sleep wellbeing: Maddie rated herself as a *three* on sleep. Her sleep onset was improved with the use of paced breathing and imagery at bedtime, but she still reported recurrent nights of fragmented sleep.

Social/relationship wellbeing: She rated herself as a *four* on relationships and social engagement. She felt an increased sense of forming a team with her husband, working together for her health and lifestyle, and reported some initial increases in contact with local friends.

Spiritual wellbeing: Maddie rated herself as a *four*, much improved in spiritual areas, yet still searching spiritually.

Illness self-management: She rated herself as a *five* on illness self-management. She experienced herself as continually active and engaged in improving her lifestyle and wellbeing.

Readiness for change: Maddie rated herself as a *five* on readiness for change. She was proud of the most dramatic period of self-directed change in her life, and still setting new goals.

Figure 6.2: Maddie's final Pathways self-assessment

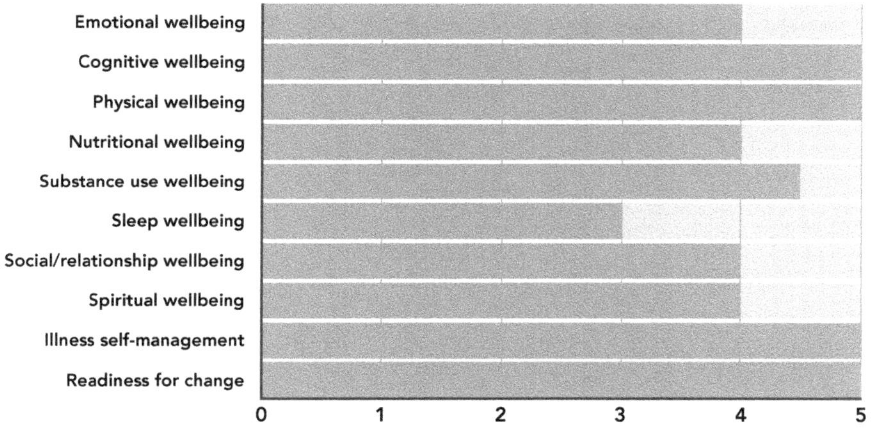

Category	Rating
Emotional wellbeing	4
Cognitive wellbeing	5
Physical wellbeing	5
Nutritional wellbeing	4
Substance use wellbeing	4.5
Sleep wellbeing	3
Social/relationship wellbeing	4
Spiritual wellbeing	4
Illness self-management	5
Readiness for change	5

Conclusion

Cancer is an unpredictable illness and Maddie's diagnosis of carcinosarcoma was concerning. She recognized that relapses are common. She was determined to remain engaged in her health and her healthcare, using both self-care and lifestyle to sustain her wellbeing as much as possible.

> **Final message:** *Making small but persisting changes in lifestyle and behavior can have positive effects throughout one's life, despite a long-term health condition. Paced breathing, guided imagery, physical activity, and nutritional changes can all aid one in managing the distress that comes with illness. Combining lifestyle changes and spiritual awakening with professional therapies can enable one to heal old traumas and discover a new sense of purpose in life. For Maddie, immersion in nature, especially taking walks in nearby dunes, was part of her personal and spiritual renewal.*

Resources

Childre, D., Martin, H., & Beech D. (2011). *The HeartMath solution* (reprint edition). HarperOne.

HeartMath Institute (2021). emWave Pro®. Available at: https://store.heartmath.org/emWave-PC/emwave-pro.html (accessed September 2024).

Katz, R., & Edelson, M. (2017). *Cancer fighting kitchen: Nourishing, big flavor recipes for cancer treatment and recovery* (2nd edition). Ten Speed Press.

Naparstek, B. (2009). A meditation to support a healthy immune system. (Audio MP3). Hay House. Available at: www.healthjourneys.com/audio-library (accessed September 2024).

Naparstek, B. (2010). A meditation to help you with radiation therapy. (Audio MP3). Health Journeys. Available at: www.healthjourneys.com/audio-library (accessed September 2024).

Naparstek, B. (2022). A meditation to help you fight cancer. (Audio MP3). Hay House. Available at: www.healthjourneys.com/audio-library (accessed September 2024).

Chapter 7:
Dealing with difficult relapses and setbacks (headache)

Summary: Successful management of a long-term condition can be difficult and time consuming. When headaches are under good control, the person follows the regimen and expects good health to continue. In the case of Angela, changes in lifestyle and job hours brought about a change in one of the parameters that affected that illness. Her headaches had been managed with a combination of medication and therapy. Then Angela's sleep became disrupted and she became sleep deprived because of new responsibilities in a job that she loved. Adequate sleep and a consistent schedule of rest and eating are hallmarks of control of migraine headache. The relapse and the accompanying psychological distress caused by the physical pain created a sense of defeat and failure.

Angela was tortured by the decision to give up the man she loved or her dream job. Pathways Levels One and Two helped her to re-establish her restorative sleep, improve her nutrition, and manage the increased job responsibilities. In Level Three, restructuring negative beliefs about herself and regaining confidence in her ability to manage stress led to a re-establishment of control of her headaches.

Keywords: migraine, resilience, positive psychology, sleep

Healing theme: navigating relapses and setbacks

The healing theme of this chapter, simply stated, is that a relapse of pain or any chronic illness can occur after a long period of good control. The return of symptoms is not a personal failure, or the fault of the care providers. Headache is a very complicated medical and psychological disorder with multiple possible triggers. The relapse of previously controlled migraine headache can occur because one of the parameters related to the headache changes. For example, travel over multiple time zones, perhaps required by the person's job, a move to a noisier neighbourhood which disrupts sleep, and increased arguments with a partner causing emotional distress, can all interfere with previously established management of headaches.

> *"The healing theme of this chapter, simply stated, is that a relapse of pain or any chronic illness can occur after a long period of good control. The return of symptoms is not a personal failure, or the fault of the care providers."*

Angela's relapse not only brought back the severe head pain; her mind was also flooded with previously held beliefs about her own failures in controlling the pain and her anger at being "forced" to lay in bed in the dark, waiting for the pain to pass. It follows then, that the healing process must be physical, emotional, behavioral, and cognitive. Through the Pathways program, Angela re-established a regular sleep schedule, healthier food choices, and increased physical activity. She learned relaxation strategies to decrease her stress reactions. Pathways Level Three connected Angela with her deep-seated anger at herself. Angela transformed her perceptions of stressful situations from "terrible" to more neutral interpretations. Finally, she recognized and accepted her true resilience in surviving so many onslaughts of pain.

Introducing Angela

During her first menstrual cycle, Angela developed a migraine that lasted three days. The pain was accompanied by nausea, several episodes of vomiting, and sensitivity to light and sound. Her mother gave her painkillers and consoled her, saying that there was a family history of migraine in the women in the family and they would get through it. After that first headache and continuing into her twenties, Angela experienced migraine with every menstrual cycle. The severity of the headaches varied; sometimes the pain was mild where she could maintain function, but at other times she was incapacitated. Angela perceived her headaches as a personal defeat. For her, every headache was a signal that she failed to cope once again. Later she would feel anger and experience frustration, become irritable with others, and overreact to minor annoyances. Her friends described Angela as "ouchy" at certain times of the month.

> *"After that first headache and continuing into her twenties, Angela experienced migraine with every menstrual cycle. The severity of the headaches varied, sometimes the pain was mild where she could maintain function, but at other times she was incapacitated."*

Angela found an expert in the treatment of headaches who practiced in a major medical centre. Through months of testing, and trials of several preventative and acute medicines, control of the headaches was achieved. Angela also sought a psychotherapist to work on her reactions to the headaches, in particular her self-blame and anger whenever she experienced an incapacitating headache.

Angela's background

Angela was the third daughter of two parents who lived in a mid-sized city. Angela's home life was stable. Her parents instilled a healthy sense of responsibility for schoolwork and chores at home. The kids were encouraged to try out different sports, musical instruments, or art, and then stay with the one activity they enjoyed. Angela participated in soccer and softball but had little natural ability for these sports. She loved being outside, regardless of the weather. Other kids complained of being too hot, too cold, or too wet, but not Angela. She became fascinated with weather patterns. When play was stopped because there were threatening black clouds, Angela did not want to take shelter, but tried to guess how bad the storm would be. At home, she did not hide when there was a storm, but instead looked out the window, riveted by the show that nature was putting on.

Chapter 7: Dealing with difficult relapses and setbacks (headache)

Angela's required school science projects were always about weather. In high school, she took pictures of cloud formations and then matched them to the weather forecast. She calculated the per cent correct forecasting of rain depending on the clouds. During college, Angela took science classes, including meteorology, and did well in all of them. She got a part-time job at the university's radio station and started doing some rudimentary weather reports. She explained threatening weather clearly, translating the national forecasts into simple terms. Few college students actually pay even minimal attention to the weather forecasts! But after a year at the station, Angela got permission to compile information that was useful to the students and present it in an interesting format. She highlighted the forecast for the upcoming outdoor sporting events and art shows and even described the best days for romantic walks in the park. "Angela's forecast" became legendary on campus.

After graduation, Angela applied for many jobs at local radio and TV stations, but it took more than a year before she had an opportunity. She would not be on the air, but would support the chief meteorologist who was a legend in weather forecasting. The chief had spent twenty years in the air force as an aviation meteorologist, and after retirement, he came to the TV station in his hometown. Angela spent her early days at the station studying weather patterns, wind velocities, and temperatures from all over the world. She had three computer screens, constantly in motion with multicolored graphs, diagrams, and calculations. Gradually, she was given more responsibility for compiling data. All information from Angela and the other staff was funnelled to the chief who was the main TV personality. She had most weekends off – unless there was a storm forecast – then no one went home.

Angela had a boyfriend, Vince. They had been together since college and cared deeply for each other. They talked about eventual marriage and having a family. But they wanted to get established in their careers and save money for a down payment on a home. After two years on the job, Angela believed her job was stable and they started talking about getting engaged. Life was good!

The local school district often requested a tour of the station or specifically a tour of the "back room" where the weather forecasts were put together and the studio where the forecast was broadcast. The station manager wanted to grant those requests, but privately complained that the kids were unruly, asked so many questions or were silent and it was not a pleasant experience. Since Angela was the most recent hire, the school groups became her responsibility. She was the contact person, set up the tours and worked on them by herself. Her gift for explaining things in a simple manner – understandable to grade-school children and stimulating for bored high-school students – garnered praise in letters and phone calls to the station by school administrators.

The chief meteorologist noticed the attention that Angela's tours had attracted, and he wanted to highlight Angela's ability to explain the weather in a simple, interesting way. He asked Angela to develop a special segment directed towards teens and middle school children. It was to be aired twice a week close to dinner time when many families would be together. Angela loved this assignment and worked hard on the presentations. Within a month, this segment was a fixture for the network.

Angela had completed three years on the job when another opportunity came her way. One of the on-air weather forecasters resigned to take a job in a larger market. Angela was asked to apply and got the job. She would not be on daily but would continue her good work in the back room, with school groups and the special forecasting for the young audience. Her shift was early morning, so she had to be at the station at 4 am to prepare for the 6 am weather forecast. Angela was ecstatic. She told Vince that this was her dream job. "I want to be the person to keep people calm in storms, but also to get them to respect nature and its powers. Nature is *awesome* and beautiful, whether it is sunny or stormy."

Within six months, the "dream job" had created irregular sleep, increased consumption of caffeine, more fast food, and overall, a very irregular schedule. Angela started to notice occasional headaches and then more severe migraine-like symptoms. Then she experienced a different type of headache. Her neck muscles felt stiff and sore, and her forehead felt like she had a tight band around it. She woke up in the morning with pain in her jaw and clenched teeth. She had less and less time to spend with Vince because she was either trying to catch up on sleep or dealing with a headache. Vince suggested that Angela return to the expert neurologist, but she refused, saying that he had spent two years testing different medicine combinations and she was not going back to him admitting failure.

Vince became more and more worried about Angela and was also concerned that she would break up with him and he would lose her. He suggested a program called Pathways that did not initially involve medical or psychiatric services. One of his co-workers had gone through the Pathways program and no one had changed his medication. He assured her that no one would change Angela's medicines without her permission.

Understanding migraine and tension-type headaches

There are many different types of headaches, and most people experience occasional head pain due to tension, overuse of alcohol, food sensitivity, or lack of sleep. When headaches become more than "occasional", occurring several times a month or causing disruption in normal functioning, the headaches are labelled chronic. The most common types of chronic headaches are migraine and tension-type headaches. Tension-type headaches may be caused by jaw clenching, intense concentration, frowning, poor posture, eye strain, missed meals, and sleep disruption, and are often associated with anxiety disorders or clinical depression. Tension headaches are described as an ache, or tightness across the forehead, in the back of the neck, around the whole head or the jaws. Tension-type headaches (TTH) usually occur more frequently than migraine; sometimes, the person may experience daily or constant pain on both sides of the head.

> *"The most common types of chronic headaches are migraine and tension-type headaches. Tension-type headaches may be caused by jaw clenching, intense concentration, frowning, poor posture, eye strain, missed meals, and sleep disruption, and are often associated with anxiety disorders or clinical depression."*

Migraine headaches are commonly throbbing and are experienced on one side of the head in the temporal or frontotemporal areas (the side of the head). Many physical disruptions co-occur with migraine, including nausea and fatigue during the headache, and in some people, the pain is preceded by the "aura", which may involve visual, auditory, olfactory (smell), or unusual bodily sensations. Current research posits that the central nervous system of migraine patients is more sensitive to changes in temperature, daily schedule, hormones (in women), stress, certain foods, alcohol, or inadequate sleep. Their brains are highly reactive, and pain occurs when a trigger starts a chain of activity in nerve cells responsible for the experience of pain. The reader is referred to the websites and printed materials listed at the end of this chapter for detailed information on migraine triggers. It is appropriate, however, to explain the role of stress in migraine or tension-type headaches.

> *"Migraine headaches are commonly throbbing and are experienced on one side of the head in the temporal or frontotemporal areas (the side of the head)."*

Stress is a common occurrence in everyday life. Work piles up, the boss is in a bad mood, the neighbours have loud parties, a bill needs to be paid when money is tight. A person's reaction to these events is defined by how they perceive the situation and how they assess their own capacity to cope. Some people do seem to have very frequent stressful situations, while others either are in fewer stressful situations or have stronger coping skills. If the person views a situation as very demanding but does not believe that it is manageable, then a stress response occurs. Everyone will be challenged by a difficult task and perhaps feel not trained or ready to meet that challenge at some times. But when a person judges most situations as overwhelming and sees himself/herself as incompetent, the risk for pain symptoms increases. In the case of tension-type headaches, posture plays a critical role. Long hours at a computer create strain on the muscles of the neck and the back and undermine the ability to relax those muscles.

Treatment of migraine

There are two main approaches to migraine care: prevent headaches before they start or stop migraines after they start.[5] Many people with migraine headaches are prescribed both acute and preventative treatments. The types of medicines comprise oral medications, nasal sprays, injections, or devices. Most medicines for migraine are prescribed by a medical provider, but over-the-counter products, such as acetaminophen or ibuprofen, can be helpful. In addition to medicines specifically designed for migraine, the provider may recommend medication more commonly prescribed for high blood pressure, seizures, depression, and anxiety. Details on the newer treatment options are beyond the scope of this book so the reader is referred to the references at the end of the chapter. Medical treatment for tension-type headaches consists of anti-inflammatory drugs, muscle relaxants, and medicines usually used to treat anxiety and depression.

> *"There are two main approaches to migraine care: prevent headaches before they start or stop migraines after they start"*

The Pathways Journey: assessment

Before setting any initial Pathways goals, Angela rated her wellbeing in the ten areas below, on a one-to-five-point scale. A score of *one* indicates very low wellbeing in an area; *five* indicates very high health status in this area:

- Emotional wellbeing
- Cognitive wellbeing
- Physical wellbeing
- Nutritional wellbeing
- Substance use wellbeing
- Sleep wellbeing
- Social/relationship wellbeing
- Spiritual wellbeing

---

5 For guidelines on both migraine prevention and acute treatments of migraine, see Pfizer (2024), www.nurtec.com/how-to-treat-migraines#preventive (accessed September 2024).

- Illness self-management
- Readiness for change

Emotional wellbeing: Angela was anxious and worried about the return of the headaches. She was angry at the headaches, like she used to be as a teenager. She was also furious at herself for slipping and now failing at controlling the headaches. She rated herself a *two*.

Cognitive wellbeing: Angela was a college graduate and was using her degree every day in her work. She felt challenged by difficult weather patterns, but not intimidated. She rated herself a *five* on cognitive wellbeing.

Physical wellbeing: Angela was active several times a week, but the activity consisted of a walk with her boyfriend and an occasional swim. Her headaches were affecting her job, her relationship with Vince, and her sense of control over her life. She rated herself a *two* to *three*.

Nutritional wellbeing: Angela was careful about foods that in her experience could trigger migraines, such as chocolate, nuts, and wine. However, she admitted that she was relying more on fast food since she was working different shifts at the station. She had increased her use of caffeine to about five cups of coffee a day. She rated herself a *three*.

Substance use wellbeing: Angela rarely drank and did not use illegal drugs. She had stopped drinking during the workup for her migraines years ago and only had an occasional beer. She rated herself a *five*.

Sleep wellbeing: Her sleep was disrupted. It took her a long time to get to sleep. She did not feel rested after sleeping and was more and more tired during the day. She rated herself a *two*.

Social/relationship wellbeing: She got along well with co-workers and had friends. She and Vince had been together for five years. Her relationships with her family of origin were good. Her self-rating was *four* to *five*.

Spiritual wellbeing: Angela prayed daily but rarely attended church. She considered herself a spiritual person and stated that her study of weather was proof that a higher power exists. Her self-rating was *four*.

Illness self-management wellbeing: This point led to a painful conversation between Angela and her Pathways team. Angela stated: "I was doing great until the last year. Now I have disgraced myself and my doctor." She rated herself a *one*.

Chapter 7: Dealing with difficult relapses and setbacks (headache)

Readiness for change: Angela was desperate. She feared that she would lose her job because the headaches would affect her work in the back room and certainly on the air. She might lose the man she loved. She said she was so ready for change but very frightened. She repeated that she did not want to contact the neurologist or let the Pathways team adjust her medicines. She rated herself a *four*.

Figure 7.1: Angela's initial Pathways self-assessment

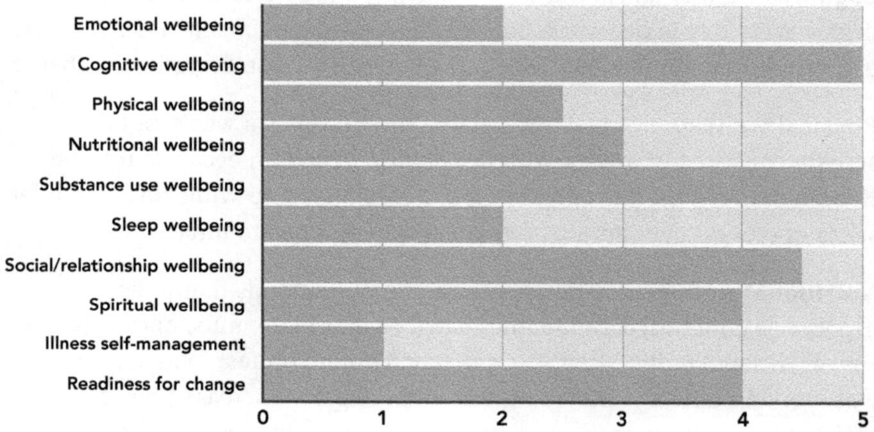

Category	Score
Emotional wellbeing	2
Cognitive wellbeing	5
Physical wellbeing	2.5
Nutritional wellbeing	3
Substance use wellbeing	5
Sleep wellbeing	3.5
Social/relationship wellbeing	4.5
Spiritual wellbeing	5
Illness self-management	1
Readiness for change	4

Pathways treatment
Level One goals
Level One involves setting goals for attainable self-directed changes, including self-care practices and simple lifestyle changes. Angela set several goals for Pathways Level One: paced slow-breath training, decreased intake of caffeine, and adjustments in mealtimes and exercise schedule.

Level One progress
Angela learned the paced slow-breathing technique quickly and started practicing several times a day. She felt calmer and noticed some relaxation of her muscles. She tried to adjust her mealtimes but was not successful. Things were often chaotic at the station and food was brought in. She recognized that some of the spicy foods made her headaches worse when she already had pain. Angela talked to the staff person who ordered the food and asked for modifications, which were provided. She tried to

decrease caffeine but was so tired and listless at certain times of the day that she needed coffee for "energy". She had increased the intensity of her exercise before Pathways, but was often active an hour before bedtime. She adjusted her exercise times to end at least two hours before bedtime.

> *"Angela set several goals for Pathways Level One: paced slow-breath training, decreased intake of caffeine, and adjustments in mealtimes and exercise schedule."*

Level Two goals

Level Two in the Pathways program includes learning specific self-care skills, often with the aid of educational materials or community resources. Angela set several Pathways Level Two goals: she committed to evaluating her posture at work, and especially to monitor her facial expressions when concentrating and looking at the computer screen. She also agreed to learn progressive muscle relaxation and adjust her sleep schedule.

Angela still spent most of her time at the computer, viewing weather data and then calculating the effects of approaching weather on her city and county. Angela asked for an ergonomic assessment and it was granted. The report stated that the desk, chair, and screens were set up perfectly, but Angela's posture was far from perfect. The behavioral specialist recommended major changes in posture. Angela was to check on her posture and break away from the screen frequently during the workday.

> *"Angela set several Pathways Level Two goals: she committed to evaluate her posture at work, and especially to monitor her facial expression when concentrating and looking at the computer screen. She also agreed to learn progressive muscle relaxation and adjust her sleep schedule."*

Angela's Pathways therapist encouraged her to learn progressive muscle relaxation (slow tense – hold – relax) and practiced with her in the office. (Appendix A includes written instructions for progressive muscle relaxation and Appendix B includes a link to a YouTube video showing the technique.)

The behavioral specialist who had specific training in sleep disorders asked Angela to keep a sleep diary of her bedtimes, the number of awakenings she experienced during the night, wake time, sleep during the day, and perception of restful sleep. He was shocked at Angela's sleep diary. Slow wave, deep, restorative sleep was minimal; dream sleep was often interrupted by an awakening. The total amount of sleep on most nights was five hours. She napped during the day between her morning shift and the evening broadcast. In addition, there had been two severe winter storms in the past weeks and the weather staff was at the station beyond their usual shifts.

Level Two progress

Angela practiced the progressive muscle relaxation exercise at least once a day and monitored her posture. The tension headaches lessened, but the migraines did not. Addressing the sleep problem was urgent since Angela reported being more and more fatigued. Melatonin was suggested to be taken one hour before bedtime and Angela was encouraged to use progressive muscle relaxation and slow breathing at bedtime. Angela also learned further "sleep hygiene" guidelines for improved sleep. The bedroom should be dark, cool, and quiet. Following these guidelines, the length of time it took Angela to fall asleep shortened, but she could not get enough sleep because of her schedule at the station. She was irritable with Vince, and he was unhappy that they did not spend much time together.

Angela came to her next Pathways appointment anxious and tearful. She had an appointment with the chief meteorologist the next day. She was sure she would be off the air and in the back room "for the rest of my life". She said that the return and worsening of the headaches had been a "catastrophe" for her career and for her relationship with Vince. "I will have to choose between the job I love and the man I love. I can't have both."

The meeting with the chief started out badly. The usually calm, pleasant, cheerful Angela was nervous, stiff, and it was obvious that she was in pain. The bright lights in the chief's office made her squint. Her jaw felt locked in place. She started to apologize for her demeanour and her recent "failings". To her surprise, the chief was kind and gently questioned her. Angela revealed her history of migraine, the good control that she had achieved, and the recent relapse. She blamed herself for all of it! She used words such as *personal disaster, catastrophe, weakness, failure,* and *disappointment*. She had not planned on telling him these details, but when he showed concern for her, it all came out. She even mentioned that she was enrolled in the Pathways program at the local medical centre. Embarrassment added to self-condemnation.

The chief had heard of Pathways and wanted Angela to continue. The next few sentences shocked Angela. The chief said:

> "This business is so hard on our health, our physical and emotional health. The person whom you replaced left for a larger market. That is true, but he also left because his mental health and his marriage were falling apart due to work pressure and the awful schedule. He took a back-room job to see if he could straighten out his life. I am not going to let that happen to you. The *kiddie weather program* is a real asset and the viewers love it. Let's expand that to five days a week. I am going to take you off the early morning weather program and put you on the noon weather. You will come to work at 10 am to prepare for noon and work until after the 6 pm broadcast."

> *"Angela's Level Three goals included re-establishing her previous sleep schedule and working on the negative, unwarranted self-criticism that she had engaged in since the relapse."*

Level Three goals

Pathways Level Three involves using professional medical, psychiatric, psychological, pastoral counseling, or other services and treatments. Angela's Level Three goals included re-establishing her previous sleep schedule and working on the negative, unwarranted self-criticism that she had engaged in since the relapse. She decided to utilize her Pathways counselor for a more intensive counseling process, focused on both sleep and self-criticism. The therapist commented to Angela:

> "You are predicting severe storms with actual possible major damage to our area. You see them coming from across the country and track them day by day and sometimes hour by hour. Sometimes, you know there could be severe damage and danger to citizens of a certain neighbourhood. You are calm on the air, professional, giving the facts, but not over-interpreting or over-doing the drama. The viewers appreciate you because you tell the truth without frightening them. The viewers believe you. The station has collected data showing that people are preparing better since you have been on the broadcast. You can apply the same mental strategies to your personal situation, predicting stress and preparing for it."

Angela rebuffed this suggestion and expressed anger at the therapist:

> "I am the failure here – I had the full workup. It took the neurologist and me two years to find the best combination of medicines. I was in therapy for eighteen months to deal with the psychological damage that the pain did to me during my high school and college years. Now everything that I treasured is gone. My schedule will be much better as soon as a replacement is found for the early morning show, but I am still the idiot and everybody at the station knows that I failed."

The therapist changed tactics. She introduced mindfulness, being in the moment, in a non-judgmental way. Her message to Angela was to practice mindful acceptance throughout her life: "Be in the moment at work; be in the moment at home as well. Spend time with Vince, accepting whatever unfolds for you in each moment." The therapist also provided a Healing Pathways Worksheet on Transforming Perceptions of Life Stress and suggested that Angela complete it and then they would review it together. (Appendix C includes the Healing Pathways Worksheets.)

The therapist also wanted Angela to check in with her neurologist even though it was several months before her scheduled appointment. Angela at first refused. The therapist mentioned that Pathways progress reports are usually sent to the participant's physicians, and the neurologist could be included in those reports. Angela saw this as a way of letting the doctor know that she was struggling without her having to tell him. She saw herself as a coward and a failure. She gave up the neurologist's name and agreed that the report could be sent to him.

Level Three progress

The chief was true to his word and Angela was pulled from the early morning news broadcast and assigned to the noon broadcast. Of course, during severe weather, no one could go home, and the meteorologists were called in on their days off. But Angela accepted this. Sleep gradually improved; the time it took her to fall asleep decreased from sixty minutes to thirty minutes. Awakenings during the night decreased to one. Angela felt more rested in the morning. Naps were eliminated. Coffee consumption decreased to two cups per day – except when there was a storm!

When the neurologist received the information from the Pathways counselor, his staff nurse contacted Angela to make an appointment for her to see him. Angela stated over and over that she was a failure and mentioned that she would not go to the appointment to have to admit her failure. The Pathways counselor contacted Vince, with Angela's permission, and he immediately agreed to go with her. The details of that appointment were never revealed to the Pathways team. But Angela returned to her next appointment, visibly calmer and more confident. Over time and with intense cognitive behavioral therapy, the negative statements about failure, catastrophe, the loss of Vince, or the loss of her job were spoken of less frequently and finally disappeared from Angela's personal vocabulary altogether.

> *"Over time and with intense cognitive behavioral therapy, the negative statements about failure, catastrophe, the loss of Vince, or the loss of her job were spoken of less frequently and finally disappeared from Angela's personal vocabulary altogether."*

Final Pathways assessment

Angela completed a final Pathways self-assessment based on the same Pathways Assessment areas as in her initial self-assessment. She rated herself on a one to five scale as follows:

Emotional wellbeing: Angela was much less anxious. She continued to work on building self-compassion and was more self-forgiving when she had a headache. She rated herself a *three* to *four*.

Cognitive wellbeing: Angela learned a new approach to thinking about the headaches through her Pathways activities. Angela now interpreted cognitive wellbeing not only as intellectual level or years of education, but how she perceived stress. She had rated herself a *five* pre-Pathways, but now with the new interpretation, she rated herself as a three working hard to get to *four*.

Physical wellbeing: Angela recognized that her physical health had improved, since the headaches were under much better control. She was still active several times a week, and she had increased the intensity of the activity. She was careful with the timing so that it would not be close to bedtime. She rated herself a *four*.

Nutritional wellbeing: Angela had returned to her previously healthy diet since the staff person at the station ordered healthy food for her. She was even more careful about foods that had triggered migraine in the past but allowed herself some leeway on her days off and on vacation. She rated herself a *four*.

Substance use wellbeing: Angela rarely drank and did not use illegal drugs. She rated herself a *five*.

Sleep wellbeing: Angela recognized that adequate hours of sleep and high-quality sleep were critical to her wellbeing, and particularly to preventing severe headaches. Her sleep was significantly improved, and she felt more rested in the morning. She rated herself as a *four*.

Social/relationship wellbeing: Angela got along well with co-workers and had friends. Her relationship with Vince was back on solid ground, and she was "waiting for the ring". She rated herself *four* to *five*.

Spiritual wellbeing: This variable was unchanged. She prayed daily but did not attend church. She continued to view nature as a sign of a higher power but did not wish to pursue these beliefs further. Her self-rating was *four*.

Illness self-management: Angela took her preventative medication as prescribed and used the acute, rescue medicine as needed. Severe migraines were rare, occurring about every six months. Severe tension headaches were also infrequent, but milder headaches occurred several times a month. Angela continued to use relaxation, mindfulness, and imagery daily, and believed that these techniques were largely responsible for her improvement. She rated herself a *four*.

Readiness for change: Angela knew that she could suffer another relapse at some time in her life. But should the migraines increase in frequency or intensity, she would be prepared to contact the treatment team, including the neurologist, and make changes as necessary. She rated herself a *five*.

Figure 7.2: Angela's final Pathways self-assessment

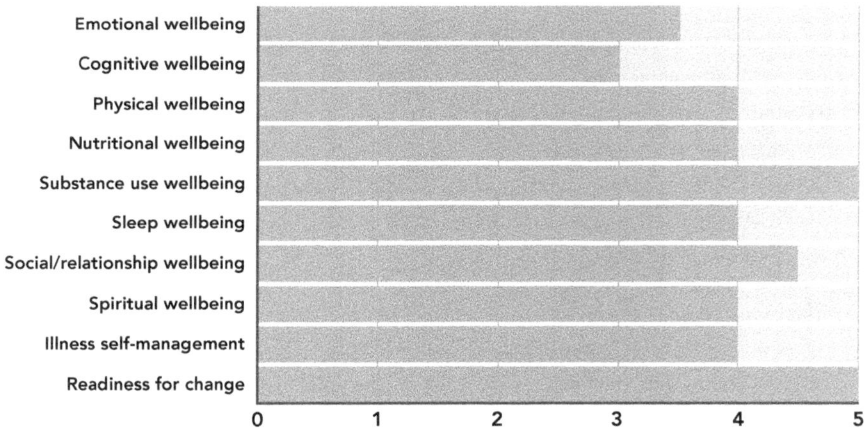

Category	Rating
Emotional wellbeing	3.5
Cognitive wellbeing	3
Physical wellbeing	4
Nutritional wellbeing	4
Substance use wellbeing	5
Sleep wellbeing	4
Social/relationship wellbeing	4.5
Spiritual wellbeing	4
Illness self-management	4
Readiness for change	5

Conclusion

This chapter highlights the challenges faced by a person during a lifelong journey with chronic headaches. In women, onset often coincides with puberty, the beginning of the menstrual cycle. Headaches may occur only monthly at first, then increase in frequency or severity. Diagnosis and management can be complex, requiring the expertise of a neurologist. The emotional pain and suffering from the headaches themselves and the disruption of life's plans and hopes can necessitate therapy sessions with a psychologist. Once control is achieved and the pain is mild and infrequent, the person assumes that this will continue long term. When a relapse occurs, self-blame, embarrassment, and disappointment can be overwhelming. This chapter has detailed Angela's journey back to good control of her headaches after a relapse that threatened her career and her relationship. All three levels of Pathways were necessary to stabilize her sleep, eating and activity schedules, and then to restructure her beliefs about the meaning of the relapse.

> **Final message:** *Relapse of symptoms of a long-term health condition, once under good control, can occur for anyone. Many chronic illnesses are known to be "relapsing and remitting disorders". Chronic conditions come and go, and symptoms worsen and improve, to the great distress of the individual. Whether pain, elevated blood pressure, or anxiety, a change in life circumstances, grief over a loss, or a move to another city can trigger a relapse.*
>
> *When this happens, it is important to retain a positive, resilient mindset. Relapse is not a personal failure. Perhaps life changes have disrupted the person's eating schedule or the usual food choices are not available. In some cases, an injury prevents the usual rigorous activity, which results in higher blood glucose values, or the arrival of a new supervisor who demands perfection and requires overtime leads to a recurrence of severe anxiety.*
>
> *In all these examples, the foundation laid through the Pathways program has not disappeared. The realistic appraisal of stress has not been "unlearned" – instead, the stress has increased. Refreshing, expanding, and intensifying the self-care skills acquired through Pathways resets the physiological and psychological control systems, the symptoms abate, and the individual recovers control.*

Resources

Macedo, D. (2021). *The sleep fix: Practical, proven, and surprising solutions for insomnia, snoring, shift work, and more*. William Morrow.

McGonigal, K. (2016). *The Upside of Stress: Why stress is good for you and how to get good at it* (reprint edition). Avery.

Peper, E., Harvey, R., & Fass, N. (2020). *Tech stress: How technology is hijacking our lives, strategies for coping, and pragmatic ergonomics*. North Atlantic Books.

Walker, M. (2018). *Why We Sleep: Unpacking the power of sleep and dreams* (reprint edition). Scribner.

Useful websites

Brain and Spine Foundation. (no date). Migraines. Available at: www.brainandspine.org.uk/health-information/fact-sheets/migraine/ (accessed September 2024).

Cleveland Clinic. (2024). Insomnia. Available at: https://my.clevelandclinic.org/health/diseases/12119-insomnia (accessed September 2024).

Cleveland Clinic. (2024). Tension headaches. Available at: https://my.clevelandclinic.org/health/diseases/8257-tension-headaches (accessed September 2024).

National Headache Foundation. (2024). Our vision: A world without headache. Available at: https://headaches.org/ (accessed September 2024).

National Institute of Neurological Disorders and Stroke. (2024). Brain basics: Understanding sleep. Available at: www.ninds.nih.gov/health-information/public-education/brain-basics/brain-basics-understanding-sleep (accessed September 2024).

Pfizer (2024). Treating migraine attacks: Breaking down migraine treatments. Available at: www.nurtec.com/how-to-treat-migraines#preventive (accessed September 2024).

Sleep Station. (2024). Sleep stages: What are they and why are they important. Available at: www.sleepstation.org.uk/articles/sleep-science/sleep-stages/ (accessed September 2024).

Web MD. (2017). How to treat a tension headache. Available at: www.webmd.com/migraines-headaches/features/treatments-tension (accessed September 2024).

Web MD. (2024). What is migraine. Available at: www.webmd.com/migraines-headaches/migraines-headaches-migraines (accessed September 2024).

World Health Organization. (2024). Migraine and other headache disorders. Available at: www.who.int/news-room/fact-sheets/detail/headache-disorders (accessed September 2024).

Chapter 8:
Recovering from loss of control, shame, and isolation (irritable bowel syndrome)

Summary: Long-term health conditions and chronic illness frequently present deep personal challenges. One's body is no longer under one's full control. Many patients experience embarrassment and shame over physical symptoms and the inability to carry out usual everyday activities. Over time, many patients with chronic conditions report less contact with friends and family. This chapter will use irritable bowel syndrome (IBS) as an example of the struggle with loss of control, shame, and isolation.

This chapter describes Brynn, a thirty-seven-year-old female accountant, who suffered severe IBS and a bewildering loss of control in her life. Her emotions ranged from shame and embarrassment to anxiety and worry to anger and bitterness. After being introduced to the Pathways Model, Brynn made a series of self-care and lifestyle changes. She was able to better manage her disorder, regain more control in her life, and improve her joy in living.

Keywords: loss of control, embarrassment, shame, isolation, irritable bowel syndrome

Healing theme: overcoming shame, embarrassment and isolation, and renewing relationships

Long-term health conditions can present a variety of challenges. One's body is no longer under one's full control. Many patients experience embarrassment and shame over physical symptoms and over uncontrollable mood swings triggered by the illness. Further, many individuals report a sense of shame over the inability to carry out usual everyday activities. Even responding to simple requests to make plans for a future date can trigger tears, because any advance planning requires predicting what one's condition will be on that specific date, which is often impossible with chronic illness. Over time, many patients with long-term conditions lose contact with once-close friends. Sometimes, even family members become impatient with the patient's inability to join in social events. Long-term illness can be a terribly lonely experience.

This chapter uses IBS as an example to illustrate both how long-term health conditions can undermine quality of life, and to show pathways to restore control, overcome shame, and reduce loneliness.

Understanding IBS

This chapter uses Irritable bowel syndrome (IBS) as an example of the struggle with loss of control, embarrassment, and isolation. IBS is a chronic bowel disorder, causing bowel tenderness and pain, with episodes of constipation and/or diarrhoea. Many individuals feel socially disabled by IBS, due to often uncontrollable bowel symptoms. Often, they progressively withdraw from activities they previously participated in and enjoyed.

IBS is a chronic functional bowel disorder. Functional means that the bowel and intestine are physically intact; there is no detectable disease process affecting the bowel, yet the bowels are not functioning normally.

IBS can be intensely uncomfortable and often painful, with tenderness or pain in the abdomen, bloating, diarrhoea, constipation, belching, nausea, and flatulence (gas). IBS is categorized by which symptoms are more frequent – diarrhoea predominant, constipation predominant, or mixed. Sometimes, diarrhoea is so frequent and uncontrollable that individuals avoid social events. Often IBS sufferers describe themselves as socially disabled, pursued by shame and embarrassment.

> "Many persons with IBS also display symptoms
> of moderate to severe anxiety, depression,
> and excessive anger. Some are diagnosed
> with emotional disorders."

Many people with IBS display symptoms of moderate to severe anxiety, sadness, irritability, and anger. Some are diagnosed with emotional disorders such as depression or panic disorder. The high levels of anxiety and other negative emotions also play a part in the vicious circle of IBS. For example, anxiety and negative emotions worsen the symptoms of IBS and worries about having an urgent need to empty the bowel and other IBS symptoms aggravate anxiety. Involving the person in self-care activities, education, and professional treatment for anxiety and emotional distress can moderate IBS symptoms.

Many persons with IBS do not seek medical care, so estimating how many people have this disorder is challenging. One researcher conducted two community surveys in the United States in the 1990s and estimated that 9% of the population developed IBS in a single year. Worldwide prevalence has been estimated as about 11% of the world population, confirming the fact that IBS is a global problem.

Introducing Brynn

Brynn was thirty-seven years old when her primary care physicians suggested she try out the Pathways Model as a self-directed program for her anxiety and "behavioral management" of IBS. Her physician had read the *Integrative Pathways* book and thought a Pathways approach might be suitable for Brynn.

Brynn was a certified public accountant. After years of hard work in bookkeeping and tax accounting, she advanced to the position of auditor. She travelled regularly to conduct audits of private companies and local government organizations. She began to struggle with intermittent diarrhoea, constipation, and abdominal bloating at about age thirty-two, and her symptoms worsened and became increasingly painful after her divorce at age thirty-five. Brynn insisted that she had accepted the divorce and adjusted to single life within the first year, but her IBS symptoms worsened over time.

Now, her fear of losing control of her diarrhoea was disrupting her work. She found herself continuously preoccupied with bowel function and the location of the closest bathroom. Her employer noticed her increasingly frequent rescheduling of auditing site visits due to more severe days of diarrhoea and recommended she get help or lose her position. She also stopped dating since she could not imagine meeting new people, enjoying an evening at a restaurant or movie, and excusing herself to run to an unfamiliar bathroom. She was overwhelmed with shame and embarrassment over her diarrhoea, and over the preoccupation with where the closest bathroom was located. Increasingly, Brynn regarded her gastrointestinal system as her enemy.

Initially, her physician attributed her bowel symptoms to work stress and it is true that her work was often stressful. But as the bowel symptoms worsened, her physician referred her to a gastroenterologist, who diagnosed IBS following the "Rome IV" medical criteria for diagnosis. Brynn suffered abdominal pain and discomfort two to three times per week. At times the pain was associated with diarrhoea and at other times with normal bowel movements or constipation. She had frequent and irregular bowel movements and frequent liquid stool. The diagnosis was IBS, mixed type, because both diarrhoea and constipation were frequent.

Her gastrointestinal (GI) specialist recommended that she reduce stress in her life, make some initial dietary changes, and take medication. She tried to reduce work stress by scheduling appointments later in the day when her symptoms were usually not as severe, but the IBS symptoms were making her work more stressful. Increasingly, the stress in her life was primarily the illness, her symptoms, and her anxiety about the next episode. At her physician's suggestion, she added more high-fiber foods, drank more water, and eliminated carbonated drinks and alcohol. The dietary changes reduced the frequency of diarrhoea slightly, but the episodes were still disruptive to her work and social life.

Brynn took over-the-counter anti-diarrheal medicines at times, mainly Imodium®, but this drug worsened her constipation, bloating, and pain. Her GI specialist prescribed additional medications for her IBS, including dicyclomine hydrochloride to reduce bowel contractions and clonazepam to address any contribution of anxiety. None of the medications seemed to have more than moderate and transient effects.

The Pathways journey: assessment

The first step for Brynn was a Pathways self-assessment. The assessment includes rating oneself from one to five in each of the ten areas listed below, with one indicating very low functioning in an area, and five indicating high levels of wellbeing in that area. In the assessment, it is also helpful to list significant strengths and weaknesses in the ten areas. Brynn rated herself in each of the ten areas. Her overall assessment is shown below:

- Emotional wellbeing
- Cognitive wellbeing
- Physical wellbeing
- Nutritional wellbeing
- Substance use wellbeing
- Sleep wellbeing
- Social/relationship wellbeing
- Spiritual wellbeing
- Illness self-management
- Readiness for change

Emotional wellbeing: Brynn experienced high levels of anxiety and depression. She saw herself as a tense, moderately obsessive person, concerned about details and performance. Those traits were virtues in her school years and in her accounting work, where attention to detail prevented mistakes. However, since her divorce and the onset of IBS, her anxiety and worry were troubling and disruptive. She was also sad and discouraged, and she found it difficult to find anything to look forward to. She often sobbed in shame and embarrassment over her episodes of diarrhoea and loss of control over her body's most intimate functions.

> *"Brynn experienced high levels of anxiety and depression. She saw herself as a tense, moderately obsessive person since childhood, concerned about details and performance."*

Chapter 8: Recovering from loss of control, shame, and isolation (irritable bowel syndrome)

Brynn completed an online anxiety scale called the Zung Self-Rating Anxiety Scale and an online depression test called the Zung Self-Rating Depression Scale.[6] On both measures, she scored in the severe range; she was severely anxious and severely depressed. For her Pathways Assessment, she self-rated herself as *one*, indicating disabling negative emotions.

Cognitive wellbeing: Brynn prided herself on being a logical, methodical person, who could apply her analytical problem solving to accounting problems and life. Now she felt less mentally alert, less focused, and more distracted. At work, she sometimes had to struggle to complete complex audits and her own financial accounts were now disorganized with overdrafts on her account and overdue notices from her credit card. This deepened her embarrassment. Brynn had always prided herself on having a first-class brain and a well-ordered life. Now, however, she rated herself as a *two*, indicating disabling disturbed thinking.

Physical wellbeing: Brynn's physical activity level was low. She had kept a dog since she was a teen, and for many years enjoyed the walking this entailed. But now her dog was in doggie daycare on workdays, so Brynn almost never walked her during the week. When the IBS symptoms were severe at weekends, she often hired a neighbour to walk her. She dreaded being caught blocks from home when her bowels acted up. She rated herself as *one* on activity, indicating severely restricted movement.

Nutritional wellbeing: As a single woman, living alone, Brynn favoured take-out food, and often chose fast food for meals and junk food for snacking. She had followed her GI specialist's advice and attempted to improve her diet, but that was stressful too, since she often spent the night in hotels when travelling for audits, and fast food was easier. She rated herself as *one* for nutritional wellbeing, indicating a severely unhealthy diet.

Substance use wellbeing: Brynn used caffeinated beverages to push through her workday when fatigued from poor sleep and pain, yet she knew that caffeine aggravated IBS symptoms. She used no recreational drugs, no addictive medications, and enjoyed a glass of wine or a cocktail about once a month when her sister visited. She rated herself as a *two* on substance use, indicating moderately unhealthy substance use, because she was aggravating her disorder with caffeine.

---

6   These self-rating scales are available on many sites online, including https://psychology-tools.com/test/zung-depression-scale (accessed September 2024).

Sleep wellbeing: Brynn identified several problems with her sleep. It took her a long time to get to sleep and then she worried about not getting enough. She woke up frequently during the night and sometimes awakened before the alarm went off. She also noticed that her mood was more anxious and troubled when she was sleep deprived and when she lacked sleep, her IBS symptoms intensified. She rated herself as a *two* on sleep, indicating poor sleep.

Social/relationship wellbeing: Brynn was often alone after her divorce. The IBS symptoms amplified her isolation, as she stayed home whenever possible, stopped dating, saw her friends rarely, and avoided social contact with co-workers. When she thought of social events, she was mortified with shame and embarrassment. Her primary social supports were a sister and two friends, who called Brynn regularly. Brynn rated herself as *two* on social wellbeing, indicating poor relationships and support.

Spiritual wellbeing: Brynn was raised in a church-going Catholic family but went through a time of shame and isolation from her previous church community after her divorce. As her IBS worsened, she stopped church attendance completely out of concern that she might experience an urgent need for the bathroom during the service. Brynn felt ashamed and guilty about her lack of religious engagement and found it increasingly difficult to pray. Yet she expressed a continued sense of faith and a yearning to re-engage spiritually. She rated herself as a *two*, indicating a poor spiritual life.

Self-management of illness and readiness for change: Brynn was a bright, take-charge person for most of her life. She was proud of managing her life as a single woman effectively before IBS, and she had followed through on many of her physician's dietary recommendations. Even though her life now was in some disarray, she wanted to manage a recovery herself. Her mother, her sister, and two girlfriends frequently offered help – to run errands or provide meals – but she refused most of this help. She read extensively about IBS online, including some medical journal articles. She was attracted to the Pathways Model and welcomed guidance in managing her disorder better. She rated herself as "desperate" and determined and ready to make any behavioral changes that would help, even if they were not convenient. She rated herself as a *three* on readiness for change, indicating preparation, because she was already gathering information about nutrition and lifestyle. She rated herself a *four* on illness self-management, indicating that she was moderately engaged in self-management.

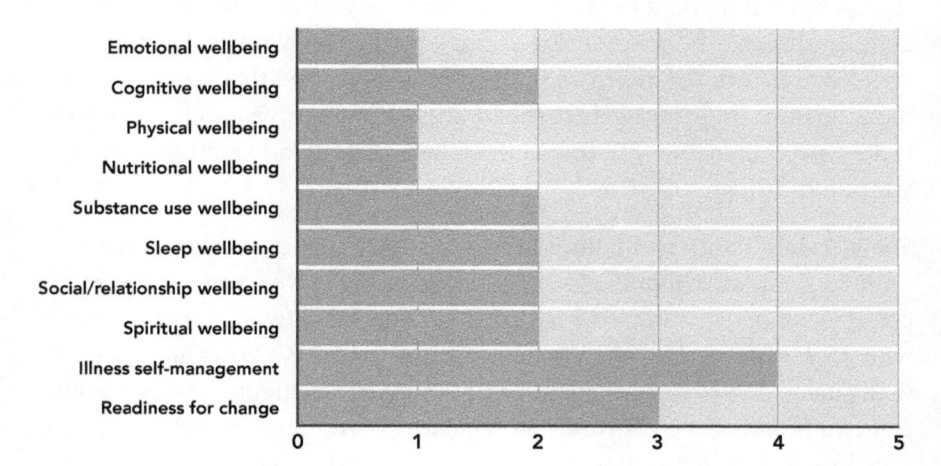

Figure 8.1: Brynn's initial Pathways self-assessment

Category	Score
Emotional wellbeing	1
Cognitive wellbeing	2
Physical wellbeing	1
Nutritional wellbeing	1
Substance use wellbeing	2
Sleep wellbeing	2
Social/relationship wellbeing	2
Spiritual wellbeing	2
Illness self-management	4
Readiness for change	3

Pathways treatment

Level One goals

Level One identifies steps that Brynn can take on her own to help herself with her IBS symptoms and her overall wellbeing. Level One goals are self-directed everyday activities that she can carry out on her own, to begin to lessen the symptoms of IBS.

Level One goal: breathing

Brynn recognized her anxiety and worry as a major contributing factor to her overall distress; she had observed that her breathing was rapid and shallow during times of worst anxiety. She had read that paced, slow breathing was useful for relaxing and quieting the mind and decided to set her first Level One goal: to practice paced, slow breathing two to three times a day, and to use slow breathing whenever she felt more anxious. She used the acronym LESS to guide her breathing exercises:

- **L** – breathe low, from the diaphragm
- **E** – breathe evenly
- **S** – breathe smoothly
- **S** – breathe slowly

She liked the acronym LESS and began using self-talk to guide herself to breathe Low, Even, Smooth, and Slow, and experience LESS anxiety with each breathing session. Brynn also practiced her LESS breathing in the parking lot before going into her office each day, and before going into any company she was auditing. She decided to practice during her lunch hour and during her afternoon break.

Initially, she was restless doing the breath exercises, but by day three she began to find that the smooth slow breathing was calming her down and her whole body felt less jittery. She felt that her diarrhoea might be getting just a little less intense as well. She also found that, with slow breathing, she could moderate her tension and calm herself when more serious episodes of anxiety occurred.

> *"Initially, she was restless doing the breath exercises, but by day three she began to find that the smooth slow breathing was calming her down and her whole body felt less jittery."*

Level One goal: nutrition

Brynn wanted to set a nutritional goal for Level One yet did not want to set a goal with a low probability of success. Her GI specialist had given her a handout of nutritional do's and don'ts for IBS, and she decided to make the following changes:

- Add high-fiber cereal to her breakfast.
- Carry a water bottle and drink cold water throughout the day.
- Eliminate carbonated beverages and alcohol for at least four weeks.

She decided to consider adding more nutritional goals if she did well with these initial goals and decided to consult a nutritionist.

Brynn felt less jittery after eliminating her caffeinated drinks, but had some difficulty staying alert. She forced herself to stand up and stretch during the workday, and when time allowed, she stepped outside and breathed fresh air. Due to the increased fluid consumption, she needed to urinate more often – but she noticed a further decrease in diarrhoea with her dietary changes.

Level One goal: sleep

Brynn decided to add one more Level One goal for herself, which was to take small steps to improve her sleep. She decided to use her LESS breathing at bedtime, to calm herself into sleep. She also committed to follow some sleep hygiene ideas. Sleep hygiene means examining both the bedroom environment and one's pre-bedtime activities for factors that may disrupt sleep. She removed her television from her bedroom and began to turn off her laptop at 9:30 pm. She was in the habit of reviewing spreadsheets of financial data while lying in bed, but she stopped this.

Brynn found that with her LESS breathing, no television, and no laptop, her sleep onset was moderately faster, and she had fewer awakenings during the night.

Level Two goals

Level Two goals continue to emphasize self-care, but draw on external assistance such as written instructions, books, phone apps, educational CDs and DVDs, podcasts, and community-based resources.

Level Two goal: breathing

For Brynn's first Level Two goal, she wanted to do more with her breathing, since it was already calming her anxious thoughts and moderating her diarrhoea. She decided to use a smartphone app called *Breathe2Relax*™ to guide her to slow and smooth her breathing further. *Breathe2Relax* is a breath pacer that guides the individual to breathe at a fixed rate chosen by the person. Brynn listened to a podcast on breathing and learned that the optimal rate of breathing for good heart rate variability and overall wellness is about six breaths per minute, so she decided to practice breathing at six breaths per minute. Heart rate variability is the moment-to-moment variation in heart rate.

> *"Brynn listened to a podcast on breathing and learned that the optimal rate of breathing for good heart rate variability and overall wellness is about six breaths per minute."*

A healthy heart is more variable, and the more variable it is, the higher the health and resilience of the person. Paced, slow breathing can increase this variability with benefits for general physical and emotional wellbeing.

Practicing her basic LESS breathing, but now with a breathing pacer set to six breaths per minute, Brynn found that she could counteract anxiety more effectively. At first, the awareness of the anxiety was troubling, but with repeated practice, she used the awareness as a positive signal that it was time to breathe.

Level Two goal: mindfulness

Brynn set her second Level Two goal as learning mindfulness. Mindfulness is a technique for remaining more fully in the present moment and accepting whatever unfolds in one's awareness in this moment, without judgment.

A community organization near Brynn's home was running a mindfulness class, so she enrolled in the class and began learning this skill. After her first two mindfulness classes, she also began to read Jon Kabat-Zinn's book about mindfulness, *Wherever You Go, There You Are*. She also ordered an educational CD from Dr Kabat-Zinn, called *Guided Mindfulness Meditation: A Complete Guided Mindfulness Program*.

Brynn found that her LESS breathing combined well with her new intention to accept the moment. The breathing slowed her mind and her body down, and she found she could watch what unfolded in the moment with more focus. She also began to practice mindfulness meditation, guided by Dr Kabat-Zinn's CD, and began each meditation session by mindfully following her breathing. She experienced a newfound sense of calm and stillness during her meditation.

Level Two goal: emotional journaling

Brynn set one more Level Two goal, to keep an emotional journal. The psychologist James Pennebaker has popularized emotional disclosure through journal writing. His research has shown that journaling can have many positive effects, including improved mood, and reduced anxiety.

Brynn followed the instructions in Dr Pennebaker's workbook, *Expressive Writing, Words that Heal*. She initially wrote whatever was on her mind and found herself spontaneously writing about her divorce and about work stress. She felt more tense and troubled as she wrote, and then a kind of release and "lightening" – somehow feeling less burdened after putting her emotions on paper. She also tried slowing her breathing when the journaling became painful, and that brought more feelings of release.

Level Two goal: reaching out from isolation

Brynn became more aware through her journaling of her sense of shame and isolation. Having diarrhoea was embarrassing and felt shameful, and she had isolated herself more and more. She completed a Healing Pathways Worksheet on embarrassment, shame, and isolation (see Appendix C for the Healing Pathways Worksheets). This led her to set a goal to reach out by phone and arrange to spend time with both her sister and a co-worker and to share the extent of her sense of shame and her sadness over isolation. She also reached out to a classmate from the mindfulness class and established regular contact with her.

Level Two progress

In summary, Brynn adopted several Level One and Two self-care behaviors and reported that her anxiety was lessened by about 50%, and her diarrhoea was a nuisance but with less frequent severe episodes. Brynn put a lot of time and effort into improving self-care and self-management. Altogether, she spent two months on Level One and three months on Level Two activities. She felt more hopeful about her life and work. She now saw her sister and her co-worker at least weekly and established a regular "phone date" with her friend from the mindfulness class. Brynn decided to move to Pathways Level Three, but to also continue attending the mindfulness class, meditating regularly, using her breath pacer set to six breaths per minute, and writing two to three times per week in her emotional journal.

Level Three goals

Brynn began her consideration of Level Three therapies with a long visit with her favourite primary care nurse. The nurse had seen her several times during the months of Brynn's Level One and Level Two activities and provided support and encouragement. The nurse even made some personal changes of her own with Brynn. She learned paced breathing from Brynn, borrowed and read the Kabat-Zinn mindfulness book, and practiced mindful acceptance in the medical office.

Brynn had reached a decision regarding her work and wanted the nurse's support. She had decided to ask for an 80% work schedule, allowing her one free day per week. Like many CPAs, she worked long work hours, and the work piled on in both corporate and personal tax season, with extra audits and tax preparation tasks. Brynn was heading into the February to April rush and wanted more time for health-supporting activities. Brynn's nurse and primary care physician wrote a brief note prescribing a four-day week for a six-month period, and Brynn's employer grudgingly accepted the change. Her boss was impressed that she was actually performing better and missing less work, and wondered why she needed to cut down now, at the busiest time of the accounting year. But he wanted her to make as full a recovery as possible, long term, so he agreed. This work reduction allowed her to better consider adding some new therapies while continuing her current self-care.

Level Three therapy: gut-directed hypnotherapy

Olafur Palsson, a psychologist/researcher in the Digestive Diseases Division at the University of North Carolina at Chapel Hill has developed a hypnosis script that is extremely effective in reducing IBS symptoms. Medical research shows that when hypnosis practitioners follow the Palsson hypnosis scripts word for word, 80% of patients show significant reductions in symptoms. The Palsson hypnosis scripts are highly soothing and relaxing; they include a broad range of imagery involving the intestines being soothed, comforted, coated, and protected from disturbance.

Brynn's GI specialist referred her to a psychologist, certified in hypnosis, who knew and used the Palsson hypnosis scripts for IBS patients. Brynn committed to attend seven hypnosis sessions following the Palsson scripts, supplemented by home practice guided by audio recordings of the therapist guiding her in a home hypnosis script. She used her LESS breathing as she began each session, combining the breath-mediated relaxation with the hypnotic effects.

She found her bowels responding to the hypnosis sessions, with less gas, nausea, bloating, and reduced frequency of diarrhoea. In addition, her anxiety was already lowered by her breathing practices and mindfulness, but now was further reduced by hypnosis. She looked forward eagerly to additional sessions and more relief. IBS patients frequently verbalize "hating their bowels" and sometimes "wanting to have them cut out". Palsson's hypnosis intervention facilitates the person's acceptance of their GI system with its flaws, and emphasizes the need to calm and comfort it.

Level Three therapy: functional medicine assessment

Brynn's primary care nurse provided a referral to a wellness clinic, an hour's drive from her home, and directed by a physician with training in functional medicine, integrative medicine, and internal medicine. The advantage of functional medicine is that it uses lab tests to develop a nutritional program individualized for the specific individual.

At the clinic, she underwent a thorough laboratory screening, aided by blood, urine, and stool samples. The physician agreed with the dietary changes she was already making but encouraged her to make several additional changes. He informed her that many but not all people with IBS did better with fewer foods that are called FODMAPS foods, such as certain vegetables (artichokes, asparagus, beans, cabbage, cauliflower), fruit (apples, apricots, blackberries, cherries, mango, nectarines, pears), and dairy products. Initially, he recommended no dairy, a low- or no-gluten diet, and gradually increasing the amount of soluble fiber in her diet. He wanted to monitor her reactions to these initial changes, before proposing further changes. He also prescribed a probiotic and two dietary supplements, and suggested peppermint tea to relax her and soothe her bowels.[7]

> *"The advantage of functional medicine is that it uses lab tests to develop a nutritional program individualized for the specific individual."*

Brynn followed the functional medicine recommendations and began packing a cooler for her travel days. If she ate food from home for breakfast and lunch, she was generally able to selectively order from a menu and stay on her program with dinner in a restaurant. She observed further normalization of her bowel frequency and consistency and became increasingly encouraged. She liked the peppermint tea and experienced the calming of her GI system when she drank it.

Level Three therapy: Acceptance and Commitment Therapy

Brynn was puzzled by her own emotions at this stage, and engaged in several long heart-to-heart talks with her hypnotherapist and her primary

---

[7] Dietary supplements in functional medicine are specifically chosen because of the laboratory analysis of sensitivities and deficiencies. Brynn's supplements are not named here because they are not recommended for all patients.

care nurse. Brynn could see benefit from most of the self-care and therapies that she was following in her Pathways program. Yet she found moments of bitterness and anger at life and God. She was thirty-seven, alone, now working restricted hours, and engaging in a huge amount of therapeutic work. Yet she saw friends and her sister living carefree lives, not having to live with so much planning or forethought. Even though she recognized the significant improvements that she had made, her anger was troubling.

She wanted to achieve more mindfulness and acceptance of where she was at, and she feared she would sabotage her own progress. Her hypnosis practitioner suggested Acceptance and Commitment Therapy (or ACT), a therapy based on a radical acceptance for each moment, with an emphasis on a self-compassionate acceptance of oneself.

Brynn completed her hypnosis program and then accepted a referral to an ACT therapist. She found that now she was struggling with spiritual questions – issues of "why me" centred on her divorce, her single status, and her long bout with illness and pain. She found herself asking long-term questions about whether her current career brought enough fulfilment, and she began to consider new relationships. She felt the emphasis on acceptance in her ACT therapy was working for her, helping her to reach more acceptance for parts of her life beyond her control.

Level Three progress

On the positive side, Brynn's IBS symptoms continued to fade, with only mild and manageable diarrhoea, mild discomfort, and no abdominal pain. She followed her functional medicine physician's guidance, and she was able to add back in some wheat and FODMAP vegetables in low quantities without relapse. She committed to continue breath work, meditation, and journaling, long term, along with some self-hypnosis that she had learned from her hypnosis sessions. She discovered that ACT therapy had paradoxical positive effects for her. ACT encourages the individual to accept anxious thoughts as they emerge, but with acceptance, her anxious thoughts lost their sting and intensity. She described this as being "less worried about my worries".

Bryn now felt less embarrassment and more acceptance about occasionally needing the bathroom at work. The realities of her IBS episodes seemed less shameful: "I found myself forgiving my bowels for their lapses. Like they were sending me an existential message to breathe, slow down, and accept; they were not attacking me." She reported a new level of comfort with her co-workers and increased time spent with old and new friends.

Final Pathways assessment

Bryn completed a final Pathways self-assessment based on the same Pathways Assessment areas as in her initial self-assessment. She rated herself as follows:

Emotional wellbeing: She rated herself as a *four*, with improved acceptance for her current life and condition, and more frequent laughter and joy.

Cognitive wellbeing: She rated herself a *four*, as she was now thinking more clearly and working more effectively, but with reduced hours.

Physical wellbeing: Brynn rated herself as a *three* on physical wellbeing. She was slowly increasing her activity and felt less frightened of bowel symptoms during activity.

Nutritional wellbeing: She rated herself as a *four* on nutrition. She had made much progress, implementing functional medicine guidelines.

Substance use wellbeing: She rated herself as a *four* on substance use. She now used minimal amounts of alcohol with only occasional caffeine intake.

Sleep wellbeing: Brynn rated herself as a *three* on sleep. Her sleep onset was improved with the use of paced breathing and imagery at bedtime, but she experienced recurrent nights of fragmented sleep.

Social/relationship wellbeing: She rated herself as a *four* on relationships and social engagement. She reported increased contact with her sister, a co-worker, and her new friend from the mindfulness class.

Spiritual wellbeing: She rated herself as a *four*, much improved spiritually, and much less troubled by thoughts of anger at God.

Illness self-management: Brynn proudly gave herself a *four* on illness self-management. She felt firmly engaged in several self-directed lifestyle choices.

Readiness for change: Brynn rated herself as a *four-and-a-half* on readiness for change because she was now successfully implementing several lifestyle goals.

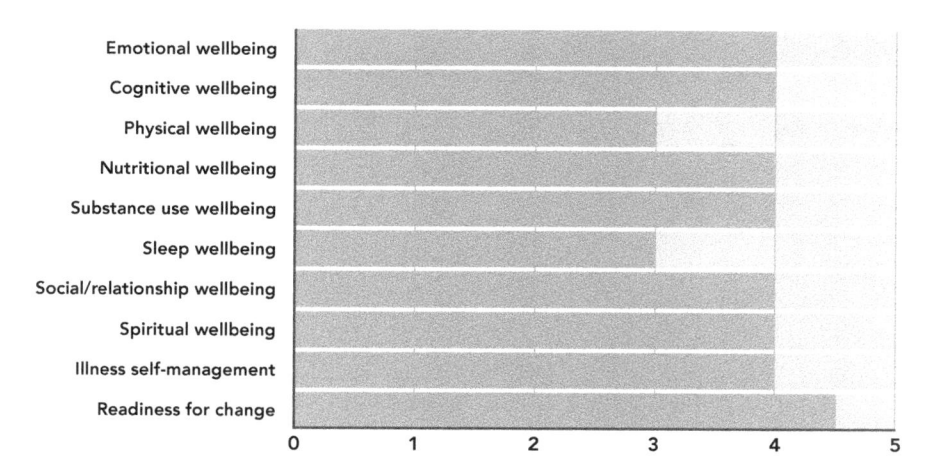

Figure 8.2: Brynn's final Pathways self-assessment

Category	Score
Emotional wellbeing	4
Cognitive wellbeing	4
Physical wellbeing	3
Nutritional wellbeing	4
Substance use wellbeing	4
Sleep wellbeing	3
Social/relationship wellbeing	4
Spiritual wellbeing	4
Illness self-management	4
Readiness for change	4.5

Conclusion

Brynn is typical of many people who benefit from introducing self-care and lifestyle changes into their life. She had the benefit of a supportive primary care physician and nurse who encouraged self-care and her active role in managing her condition. She experienced more relief from her particular illness than many do, although she accepted that individuals with IBS can relapse, and she might have to resume her self-care more aggressively in future. She gained more acceptance and forgiveness for her body, and even her bowels, no longer experiencing them as "enemy organs". Through her Pathways program and its emphasis on a mind-body-spirit approach, she learned to not only manage her condition but to thrive. Now that Brynn is much healthier physically, she is able to consider the universal challenge of finding her way in life.

Final message: *Becoming personally involved in one's health and wellbeing pays dividends. Making self-directed changes can restore a sense of control over one's life. People with IBS and many other long-term conditions can reduce the emotional suffering of living with a disease and improve their quality of life. For some, lifestyle changes and new self-care practices will also reduce the frequency and intensity of physical symptoms.*

Resources

Kabat-Zinn, J. (1994). *Wherever You Go, There You Are: Mindfulness meditation in everyday life.* Hyperion.

Pennebaker, J. W., & J. F. Evans (2014). *Expressive writing: Words that heal.* Idyl Arbor, Inc.

Chapter 9:
Managing pain, recovering activity, and improving mood (osteoarthritis)

Summary: Many long-term health conditions are accompanied by significant pain, and individuals with long-term or recurrent pain frequently avoid everyday activities that aggravate pain. Pain and avoidance of activity affect both job and home life. Over time, many people with chronic pain become sedentary, more isolated, and depressed. This chapter will use osteoarthritis of the hand to illustrate the effects of pain and pain avoidance on both functionality and quality of life.

The article introduces Margaret, a fifty-five-year-old technical writer with osteoarthritis in the left hand to illustrate the challenges of living with pain. Initially, Margaret's pain was intermittent and moderate, but over time it grew intense and chronic, aggravated by a wide variety of everyday activities. As she attempted to avoid activities that worsened the pain, her life became more limited and emptier with increases in both depressed mood and anxiety.

> Margaret pursued a self-directed Pathways Model plan, to increase self-care and introduce changes in her lifestyle. She benefitted from an integrative program of pain-management activities, including occupational therapy, acupuncture, hypnosis, and spiritual counseling. She was able to resume several leisure time activities and recover the zest of her previous life.
>
> **Keywords:** arthritis, pain, avoidant behavior, Pathways Model, palliative care, lifestyle change

Healing theme: experiencing pain, avoiding activities that intensify pain, and recovering an active and rewarding life

Many long-term illnesses and conditions are accompanied by pain, including back injuries, headaches, cancer, fibromyalgia, neurogenic pain, and arthritis. Approximately one-quarter of adults report at least intermittent pain, and in many the pain is constant. Long-term pain is more frequent in older adults.

Frequently with pain comes pain avoidance – the individual avoids activities that worsen pain. A vicious cycle develops in both mind and body. The inactivity triggers muscular deconditioning and secondary muscular pain. The narrowing of everyday life and diminished engagement in rewarding activities frequently give rise to depression and a deep sense of loss. Depression may be intermittent and moderate, but for some the depression becomes severe and disabling.

> *"The greatest evil is physical pain."*
> (Saint Augustine)

This chapter will use osteoarthritis as an example of a pain-provoking disorder and present the case narrative of Margaret, a fifty-five-year-old technical writer with osteoarthritis of the hands. Guided by the Pathways Model, Margaret used self-care, lifestyle change, and non-pharmacological therapies to recover rewarding activities and joy in her life.

Understanding arthritis and osteoarthritis

Arthritis refers to a family of disorders, involving disease, pain, and inflammation in the joints of the body. Arthritis symptoms include swelling, pain, stiffening, and limited range of motion in a joint. According to the Centers for Disease Control and Prevention (CDC), approximately one-fourth of adults in the United States have been diagnosed with arthritis, and that prevalence increases with age. Among adults with arthritis, over 40% report arthritis-related limitations in their activity. The Belgian medical researcher Jean-Yves Reginster described the global magnitude of arthritis suffering, constituting both an economic burden and an impact on quality of life worldwide. He emphasized that the percentage of the populace suffering from arthritis is increasing, along with the ageing of the world population.

The most common types of arthritis are osteoarthritis (OA), autoimmune inflammatory arthritis (including rheumatoid arthritis), and infectious arthritis. This chapter will focus on OA, a progressive joint disease involving the breakdown of joint cartilage. OA most commonly affects the hands, the spine, the knees, and the hips. OA can develop after an injury, such as a fracture, it can develop from physically demanding work, or it may stem from lifestyle factors, such as being overweight, lack of exercise, or poor nutrition.

OA in the hand is a highly prevalent disease affecting about 10% of the general population. The thumb's carpometacarpal joint is among the sites most frequently affected. OA in the hand causes pain, stiffness, impaired physical function, lower quality of life, and distress over the appearance of the hand. In some patients, the impact of the disease is as severe as rheumatoid arthritis. Currently, OA is the most rapidly increasing form of disability worldwide. Osteoarthritis is a significant factor, along with overall frailty, undermining independent living.

Currently, no medical treatments appear to reliably modify OA, and patients frequently draw on complementary and alternative therapies to assist in managing their condition. Medical research shows at least moderate support for several non-surgical, non-pharmacologic interventions, including physical therapy (PT) and occupational therapy (OT), lifestyle modification, and several complementary and alternative therapies. Many of these therapies can be used in combination with medication for inflammation and pain.

137

Introducing Margaret

Margaret was a technical writer for an office furniture manufacturer. She spent a good part of each day at a computer keyboard, drafting explanatory text about her company's modular office systems, and reviewing and editing both product-design and product-marketing materials. Margaret had attended an engineering school and earned a dual major in design engineering and technical writing. Her background made her useful in her company, where she often served as a bridge between customers and the company design and production divisions.

Margaret was married to an estate-planning attorney, who was supportive of her career and empathetic to her concerns when pain developed. Margaret and her husband had two daughters, both in college and rarely home.

The onset of Margaret's arthritis pain came at weekends, not at work. She was an avid card player, and frequently spent Saturday evenings playing bridge with her husband and several friends. In her late forties, she began to experience left-handed pain, especially in her thumb, when shuffling cards. Short term, she managed the pain by asking others to take her turn shuffling. Then she developed a different way to shuffle with her fingers, not placing pressure on her thumbs.

Over time, the left-handed pain began to occur at work, during prolonged sessions of working on a keyboard. She found some relief with an over-the-counter analgesic (a non-steroidal anti-inflammatory medicine). Initially, Margaret's pain was intermittent and moderate, but over time the pain grew intense and persisting, aggravated by a wide variety of once-normal activities. She increasingly avoided anything provoking pain and gave up many of her favourite pastimes and sources of joy. She continued to work, but her avoidance of left-handed typing and similar activities limited her efficiency. Margaret experienced a depressed mood, a profound sense of loss for her life as it had once been, and anxiety about not living up to expectations in the workplace.

Finally, at age fifty, she reported growing pain to her primary care physician, who referred her to a rheumatologist, a specialist in musculoskeletal and inflammatory diseases. The rheumatologist conducted blood work, joint fluid samples, x-rays, fMRI imaging, and a thorough history. The x-rays showed moderate bone damage and a narrowing of joint spaces in both hands, worse in her left hand and in the left thumb carpometacarpal joint. The fMRI showed only mild damage to the soft tissue in the left hand. There were no indications of causes for the pain other than probable OA. The rheumatologist prescribed an anti-inflammatory medication and an over-the-counter topical cream to alleviate pain. He also provided a handout of hand exercises to maintain range of motion. Her condition improved slightly with the medication and topical cream, then gradually worsened over time. She attempted the hand exercises several times and then discontinued them due to pain.

Margaret was fifty-four years old when her neighbour, a nurse, suggested she try the Pathways Model for self-care and lifestyle change, to manage her OA. The neighbour had used the Pathways Model in managing hypertension, relying especially on nutritional changes, regular meditation, and increased exercise and activity.

The Pathways journey: assessment

Margaret worked with a local health psychologist and a health coach to learn and apply the Pathways Model. The Pathways Model begins with an assessment of the individual's health status, behaviors that impact personal health and wellbeing, and medical and mental health history. Only by identifying areas of strength/resilience as well as areas of lifestyle and behavioral deficits can the individual realistically formulate a practical self-care and lifestyle change plan. Ten factors are included in the Pathways Assessment:

- Emotional wellbeing
- Cognitive wellbeing
- Physical wellbeing
- Nutritional wellbeing
- Substance use wellbeing
- Sleep wellbeing
- Social/relationship wellbeing
- Spiritual wellbeing
- Illness self-management
- Readiness for change

Margaret rated herself in each of these ten areas, on a five-point Likert-type scale, with one indicating very low functioning in an area, and five indicating high levels of wellbeing in that area. She identified particular strengths in several areas, but serious problems in others:

Emotional wellbeing: She rated herself as a *one*, because she experienced high levels of depression and anxiety.

Cognitive wellbeing: She rated herself as a *two*, because she experienced increasing inattention and difficulty with concentrating on her technical writing.

Physical wellbeing: She rated herself as a *one* on physical wellbeing, due to her avoidance of exercise and physical activity because activity aggravated her pain.

Nutritional wellbeing: She rated herself as a *five* on nutrition because her diet included predominantly healthy home-cooked food.

Substance use wellbeing: She rated herself a *five* on substance use, with no use of non-prescribed drugs, moderate alcohol use, and minimal use of analgesics.

Sleep wellbeing: She rated herself as a *two* on sleep quality, because she suffered both delayed onset and frequent awakening.

Social/relationship wellbeing: Margaret rated herself as a *five* because her relationships seemed one of her strengths, and she felt blessed with supportive friends and family.

Spiritual wellbeing: She rated herself as a *four* on spirituality. She was raised with a traditional Protestant religious background and continued to enjoy regular involvement with her church.

Illness self-management: She rated herself as a *one* on illness self-management. She had almost no sense of what she could do to manage her illness. She was ready to take action but did not know how to begin.

Readiness for change: Margaret rated herself as a *five*, because she was frustrated that the pharmacologic approach had not improved her condition. She felt more than ready to attempt alternative approaches.

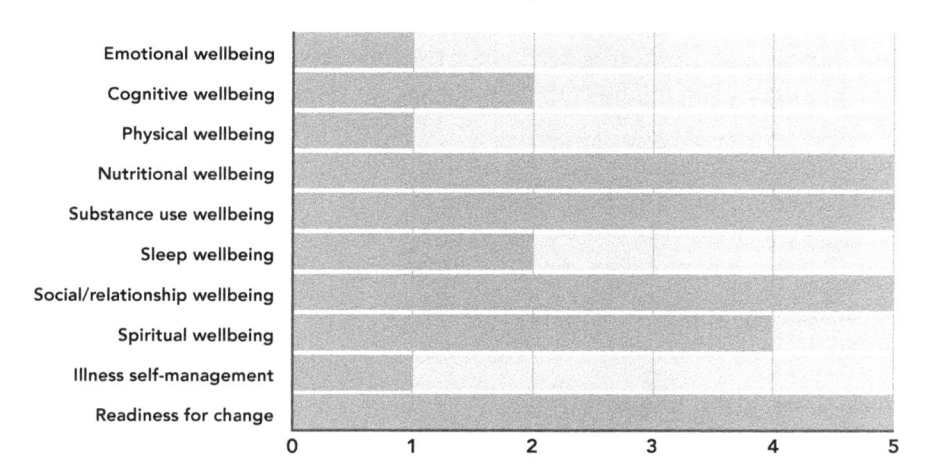

Figure 9.1: Margaret's initial Pathways self-assessment

Category	Score
Emotional wellbeing	1
Cognitive wellbeing	2
Physical wellbeing	1
Nutritional wellbeing	5
Substance use wellbeing	5
Sleep wellbeing	2
Social/relationship wellbeing	5
Spiritual wellbeing	4
Illness self-management	1
Readiness for change	1

Pathways treatment

Level One goals

In the Pathways Model, Level One activities include self-directed changes in everyday behaviors and changes in health-related lifestyle. After the initial Pathways assessment, the Pathways therapist and the patient engage in dialogue to explore possible small steps for self-directed change. Level One goals typically include adopting self-care activities and small lifestyle changes. Margaret proposed four initial Level One activities: overcoming avoidance behaviors, occupational therapy hand exercises, breathing exercises, and emotional journaling.

Level One goal: overcoming avoidance behavior

In the years after she began suffering arthritis pain, Margaret relied extensively on avoidance behaviors as a way of coping. When her rheumatologist recommended hand exercises, she tried the exercises, experienced discomfort, and stopped them. Over time, she increasingly avoided most physical activity. She experienced her life as more empty and depressing. Margaret's health coach provided her with a Healing Pathways Worksheet on "Overcoming Avoidance Behaviors and Recovering a Rewarding Life" (see Appendix C). She completed the worksheet and immediately decided to make a new approach to the hand exercises, as part of overcoming avoidance behavior.

Level One goal: hand exercises

Margaret committed herself to daily practice with occupational therapy hand exercises as recommended by her rheumatologist four years earlier. Initially, she followed the nine hand exercises recommended by the Arthritis Foundation.[8] The exercises involved: gently spreading her fingers and thumb; gently forming a fist and squeezing an exercise ball; gently forming a fist and then stretching the fingers out straight; rolling the fingers; bending the fingers and thumb toward the palms, one at a time; and other stretching motions in the hands, wrists, and fingers. The emphasis was on gentle movement and not persisting in any motion that aggravates arthritic pain.

Level One goal: breathing

Margaret suffered increasingly severe anxiety and moderate depression as her arthritis pain worsened. When she was anxious, the depression seemed to worsen. After some discussion about various strategies for coping with anxiety and stress, she decided to begin breathing exercises, using instructions available online[9]. She learned to breathe using the acronym LESS:

> **L**ow – breathing from the diaphragm
> **E**ven – breathing evenly with a consistent breath rate
> **S**mooth – breathing gently and smoothly, without effort
> **S**low – breathing at approximately six breaths per minute

She practiced breathing in through her nostrils and out through her mouth, with pursed lips. Gradually, she extended the exhale longer than the inhale, consciously releasing tension on each outbreath.

Level One goal: emotional journaling

Given her high levels of anxiety and depression, and her personal observation that high anxiety days and severe arthritis pain days ran together, Margaret chose a third Level One activity focused on her emotions. Margaret had kept a journal in past years, and often felt an emotional release after expressing her emotions on paper. She now chose to follow the guidelines of James Pennebaker, a psychologist whose extensive research showed that journaling on one's emotions can improve mood, reduce anxiety, enhance immune function, and improve overall wellbeing.

---

8 See www.arthritis.org/health-wellness/healthy-living/physical-activity/other-activities/9-exercises-to-help-hand-arthritis (accessed September 2024).

9 https://bit.ly/GentleBreathing (accessed September 2024)

Margaret's health coach gave her a copy of Pennebaker's most recent workbook, *Expressive Writing: Words that Heal*. She committed to following the workbook guidelines: dedicating fifteen to twenty minutes a day to journaling, writing about her deepest and most intense emotions, allowing herself to express herself freely, closing the journal after the set time, placing it in a drawer, and going about her day.

Level One progress

Margaret embraced the idea of reclaiming parts of her life and reducing her use of avoidance as a way of coping. She practiced her hand exercises daily for fifteen to twenty minutes. She found that some of the exercises (such as making fists) were too painful, so she limited her practice of them. However, she noticed within two weeks that the range of motion in her wrist, fingers, and thumb was greater, which encouraged her to continue the exercises. She found that, with practice, many of the exercises involving bending and extending the fingers were less painful.

Margaret had sung in a madrigal group in college, and she found the paced, gentle, diaphragmatic breathing came easily for her. She could feel her emotions calming and her musculature relaxing as she practiced her paced breathing more frequently and for longer time periods. She experimented with beginning paced breathing for ten minutes before and during her hand exercises and found she could go farther in the hand exercises if she did them in combination with the breathing. She also reported becoming more aware when anxiety and tension were coming on for her, often in conjunction with her workplace and work activities. Implementing her paced breathing whenever she sensed rising tensions often reduced her stress level. Overall, she experienced less frequent times of severe anxiety and was often able to moderate the anxiety when it occurred, using paced breathing.

When Margaret began journaling, she forgot one of Dr Pennebaker's guidelines. She wrote for over an hour on two consecutive days, became very agitated, and experienced increased anxiety and pain. Her health coach reminded her to set a time for journaling, between fifteen and twenty minutes, use a timer, and stop when she reached the specified time. Following the guidelines more closely, she began to experience a physical and emotional *lightening* with each day's journaling. She also felt less distress about her pain. She explained carefully that the pain didn't seem different, but she felt less distress about it.

Level Two goals

In the Pathway Model, Level Two includes learning self-regulation strategies and using community resources as well as online/digital resources. Margaret chose two Level Two interventions that extended her exercise and activity – aquatherapy and gentle yoga – and one that focused on psychological coping – mindfulness training. Meanwhile, she continued her Level One activity.

Level Two goal: aquatherapy

Aquatherapy (or aquatic exercise) involves engaging in a program of gentle graded exercise while immersed in a therapeutic pool, with the water usually maintained at 34°C (94°F) or higher. Immersion in warm water facilitates muscular relaxation, and at the same time moderates any impact on joints. The aquatherapy program that Margaret enrolled in was supervised by physical therapists, and the exercise regimen was designed for people with arthritis, neuropathy, and other forms of chronic pain. The program exercised the entire body, with arm, leg, and torso stretches, and included individually tailored hand exercises for Margaret, mirroring the hand exercises she was doing already, but now while immersed in the pool.

Level Two goal: gentle yoga

After six weeks in the aquatherapy program, Margaret was encouraged to begin a gentle yoga program. Gentle yoga is based on a modification of traditional Hatha yoga, with a slower pace, less intense positions, and greater emphasis on meditation, breathing, and relaxation. Gentle yoga is more accessible for individuals with arthritis and other pain conditions, and for people whose muscles are de-conditioned due to a sedentary lifestyle. Margaret enrolled in a gentle yoga program at a local community organization, conducted by an exercise physiologist.

Level Two goal: mindfulness

Mindfulness training guides the individual to a heightened moment-to-moment awareness of present events, as they unfold. The founder of the Western mindfulness movement, Jon Kabat-Zinn, described mindfulness as "paying attention in a particular way: on purpose, in the present moment, and non-judgmentally". Cultivating mindfulness frequently reduces anxiety and negative emotions, and for many people, also moderates distress over pain. Margaret initially used a mindfulness training CD to gain mindfulness skills. Later, she enrolled in a six-week mindfulness and meditation class sponsored by a local community organization.

Level Two progress

Margaret found the warm water in the aquatherapy pool soothing and discovered that many movements and exercises were less of a strain and less painful in warm water. She still experienced some difficulty making a fist with any force, and even bumping her left thumb during movement sometimes triggered sharp pain that she felt throughout her body. She was able to rest briefly and resume activity, but whenever this happened, she found herself combatting anxiety before the next aquatherapy session.

Margaret enjoyed her initial yoga sessions but found herself wishing she could do them in warm water. Some of the yoga positions (asanas) were challenging and painful for her, and she found herself trying to modify her position and eliminate pressure on her hands. At this time, she asked whether she could begin acupuncture or some other Level Three therapies then under discussion, in hopes that this would help her engage in yoga with less discomfort.

Margaret found the mindfulness approach attractive and began experimenting with a kind of mindful distancing from her own body and pain. She experimented with engaging in an inner dialogue with herself as she formed a fist or engaged in yoga, observing her own physical distress as though from a distance, as an external observer. Her instructor in the mindfulness class encouraged her to combine her paced breathing with her mindfulness strategies before and during her yoga sessions, and the combination seemed to help her manage discomfort in some yoga positions. She experienced the combination of breathing and mindfulness as almost magical in quieting her mind and emotions. She reported that the average intensity of both anxiety and depression was perhaps a fourth of her original emotional distress.

Level Three goals

Level Three interventions are professional therapies and treatments delivered by health professionals and other relevant professionals. This might include mainstream medicine including medication, complementary therapies such as acupuncture and Reiki, and spiritual guidance. In Margaret's case, she began two Level Three therapies during the same time in which she carried out her Level Two activities. The pain in her thumb was aggravated by increased activity including yoga, and both Margaret and her Pathways team were hopeful that Level Three interventions such as acupuncture might moderate pain and enhance her tolerance for activity.

Margaret initially selected acupuncture and occupational therapy for her Level Three treatments, along with hypnosis, with an emphasis on hypnosis for pain management.

Although she had rated herself as high in her spiritual wellbeing, in her Pathways Assessment, she now also asked for help in formulating some kind of Level Three spiritual intervention. Margaret grew up in a Protestant family, with regular church attendance and church-sponsored youth groups. She continued to attend a local Episcopal church with her husband. Yet she found herself angry with God over the impact of pain on her life and work, alternating with questioning whether she had caused her suffering by past inattention to spiritual matters. On good days, she dismissed the self-blame as nonsense, yet it caused her significant distress. Margaret's health coach suggested she see a minister employed at a nearby retreat centre, who had a reputation for counseling many individuals with long-term medical problems.

Level Three therapy: acupuncture and acupressure

Margaret began to see a local osteopathic physician, who was also certified in acupuncture. He proposed a treatment protocol in which he would use a relatively standardized acupuncture needling and manual acupressure to acupoints on the hand and forearm, in the office. He supplemented that by teaching her acupressure techniques. Once he identified acupressure points that seemed to provide relief in the office, he taught her and her spouse to apply manual pressure to the same points at home.

Level Three therapy: occupational therapy

Margaret obtained a referral for occupational therapy (OT) from her rheumatologist. The OT initially took a detailed history of her current activities, activities that trigger pain, and medical history. She tested her hand strength and measured range of motion, and asked her to demonstrate the hand exercises she was currently practicing. She guided Margaret to modify her movements somewhat in the hand exercises. She also discussed further modifications in everyday activities to strain her thumbs less. Margaret had already designed some movement modifications to reduce pain when typing and shuffling cards.

The OT also reviewed Margaret's experience with early morning pain on awakening. Margaret frequently experienced more intense pain in the morning, worse if she lay on a hand or seemed to have twisted a hand in the night. The OT fitted Margaret with a hand splint, designed to immobilize and protect her hand at night. Finally, the OT provided cold and hot packs, and suggested she alternately apply heat and cold when the pain was more intense.

Level Three therapy: hypnosis

Margaret requested hypnosis and was referred to a local psychologist who specialized in hypnosis for pain. The hypnotist guided Margaret into hypnotic trance inductions, using gentle breathing, eye fixation, and hypnotic imagery. Margaret responded easily, displaying high hypnotic ability. Once Margaret was deeply relaxed in a trance, the therapist used a variety of pain-management strategies to modify her pain experience. He also used dissociative strategies: Margaret observed her pain from a distance and perceived it as something external, separate from herself. She felt that her mindfulness training was deepened at this point, blending with the hypnotic dissociation. As she showed benefit from specific hypnotic strategies, her therapist emphasized Margaret mastering self-hypnosis, to achieve the same hypnotic effects without the therapist.

Level Three therapy: spiritual counseling

Margaret expressed embarrassment to the pastoral counselor, even shame, at being so angry at God. The counselor disclosed some of her own experiences with cancer-related pain and her sense of angry unfairness, that God would allow her to suffer pain after she dedicated her entire life to serving Him and the church. She introduced Margaret to several other women with significant pain, each of whom struggled with religious conflicts. Margaret became more accepting of her anger. The counselor also recommended that she read a book by Rabbi Harold Kushner, *When Bad Things Happen to Good People*, which suggested a variety of ways in which people have come to terms with tragedies and challenges.

Level Three progress

Margaret experienced little benefit from her initial acupuncture and acupressure sessions and was quite disappointed. She entered her third session in intense left-handed pain. She entered the room breathing slowly and gently, using a mindful observational mode, yet still in pain. She experienced immediate relief when her acupuncturist administered manual pressure to the Baxie acupoints on the dorsum of the hand. Her acupuncturist then guided her husband to apply pressure to these same points, again providing relief. The acupuncturist also experimented with adding electrical stimulation to these points and others and provided additional relief. Margaret asked her husband to accompany her to the beginning of some of her gentle yoga sessions. She found that if he applied pressure to the same acupoints, she experienced less pain and discomfort during yoga.

Margaret appreciated her OT's careful review of the onset of her arthritis pain, her analysis of how movement affects her pain, and the review of a wide range of strategies for managing life with arthritis. Wearing a splint seemed to reduce the morning hand pain, and she believed that, overall, the pain was less severe on days after she wore the splint to bed.

Margaret saw the OT several times and carefully showed her the changes she was now making in her hand exercises. She experimented with heat and cold. She felt some slight relief from the alternating heat and cold, but not enough that she wanted to sit with the packs placed on her hands. Margaret decided to see the OT intermittently to assess her range of motion and strength over time, and for further ideas about movement and pain.

Margaret took easily to the hypnotic approach to pain and was able to engage in self-hypnosis to achieve hypnotic benefits without the therapist. She experienced two kinds of transformation in her pain. First, she was able to moderate the intensity of her pain sensation, using imagery of making it smaller, moving the pain around in her body, and moving it outside her body. Second, she found that when the pain was very intense, she could observe it as something there, apart from her, not touching her personally.

Margaret felt the intensity of her anger and shame lessen as she spoke several times to her pastoral counselor. She came to accept that negative emotions were a normal and acceptable response to pain and illness. She also came to identify specific psalms and prayers that gave her comfort in her times of continuing pain. She combined her mindfulness techniques and gentle diaphragmatic breathing with prayer for a deeper prayer experience. Margaret also agreed to participate in a monthly support group at the retreat centre for women living with long-term conditions. She benefitted from the perspective she gained from the other women's struggles and their sometimes-heroic persistence in coping.

Final Pathways assessment

Margaret completed a final Pathways self-assessment based on the same Pathways Assessment areas as in her initial self-assessment. She rated herself on a one to five scale as follows:

Emotional wellbeing: She rated herself as a *three*, with improved acceptance of her current condition, and reduced anxiety, depression, and anger.

Cognitive wellbeing: She rated herself a *four*, with enhanced attention and focus.

Physical wellbeing: She rated herself as a *three* for physical wellbeing. She was slowly increasing activity and was now able to tolerate many yoga positions.

Nutritional wellbeing: Margaret rated herself as a *five* on nutrition. She regularly implemented a dietary plan consisting of healthy self-prepared foods.

Substance use wellbeing: She rated herself as a *five*, with reduced use of analgesics, and infrequent use of alcohol.

Sleep wellbeing: Margaret rated herself as a *three* in sleep. Her sleep onset was improved with regular use of self-hypnosis and mindfulness at bedtime. However, she continued to experience frequent awakenings in the night.

Social/relationship wellbeing: She rated herself as a *five* in her relationships and social engagement. She was in regular contact with friends and family and experienced a growing openness with her support group.

Spiritual wellbeing: Margaret rated herself as a *four-and-a-half*. She felt she was healing spiritually and was now able to find comfort in prayer.

Illness self-management: She rated herself as a *four* because she was consistently engaged in several self-directed lifestyle choices, with benefits to her health.

Readiness for change: Margaret rated herself as a *five* as she was successfully implementing her lifestyle and self-care goals.

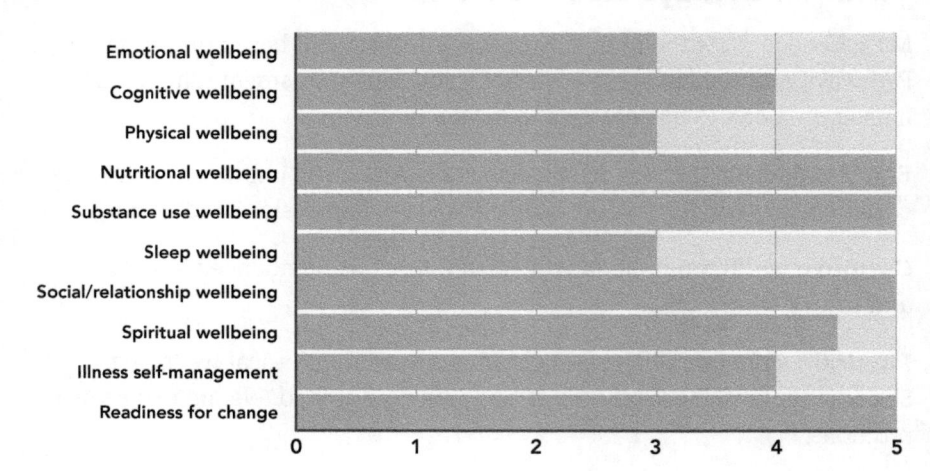

Figure 9.2: Margaret's final Pathways self-assessment

Category	Score
Emotional wellbeing	3
Cognitive wellbeing	4
Physical wellbeing	3
Nutritional wellbeing	5
Substance use wellbeing	5
Sleep wellbeing	3
Social/relationship wellbeing	5
Spiritual wellbeing	4.5
Illness self-management	4
Readiness for change	5

Conclusion

Osteoarthritis is a progressive condition. Many non-pharmaceutical interventions can provide palliative benefit (relieving symptoms without addressing their cause), and moderate the distress that accompanies OA. Lifestyle changes, notably remaining active, maintaining a normal body weight, getting adequate sleep, and managing stress and negative emotions can all moderate the severity of OA. Self-care practices and coping skills can also have palliative effects, moderating distress.

Margaret's first step in her Pathways plan was to confront the way she relied on avoidance as a way of coping. She embraced reducing her avoidance behaviors and reclaiming activities that previously brought her happiness. During the time she was in active Pathways-oriented treatment, Margaret maintained several positive lifestyle changes and continued to use several self-care practices including gentle diaphragmatic breathing, mindfulness, self-hypnosis, and self-administered acupressure.

Margaret was grateful for the self-directed aspect of her Pathways Model. At a one-year telephone follow-up, she reported continued use of many of the palliative strategies. Her anxiety was mild and her mood was stable. Her hand pain was much reduced compared to when she began treatment. Her self-care skills enabled her to cope with emotional distress and pain when they occurred. Margaret continued to remain active at home and in her career.

Final message: *Becoming active in one's own health and wellbeing pays dividends. Avoidance behaviors are a trap for people with pain or anxiety, and overcoming avoidance is key to recovering a good quality of life. Long-term conditions such as osteoarthritis are not curable, but many of the symptoms of OA and other long-term illnesses moderate with positive lifestyle changes and pain-relieving self-care. Many patients following the Pathways Model report less frequent episodes of acute distress as well as moderated intensity of pain during episodes.*

Resources

Arthritis Foundation. (no date). About arthritis. Available at: www.arthritis.org/about-arthritis (accessed September 2024).

Arthritis Foundation. (no date). Nine exercises to help hand arthritis. Available at: www.arthritis.org/health-wellness/healthy-living/physical-activity/other-activities/9-exercises-to-help-hand-arthritis (accessed September 2024).

Kabat-Zinn, J. (2005). *Wherever You Go, There You Are: Mindfulness meditation in everyday life* (10th edition). Hachette Books.

Kushner, H. (2004). *When Bad Things Happen to Good People* (reprint edition). Anchor.

McGrady, A., & Moss, D. (2013). *Pathways to Illness, Pathways to Health*. New York, NY: Springer.

McGrady, A., & Moss, D. (2018). *Integrative pathways: Navigating chronic illness with a mind-body-spirit approach*. Springer.

Pennebaker, J., & Evans, J. (2014). *Expressive Writing: Words that heal*. Idyll Arbor.

Chapter 10:
Coming out of the tunnel of despair (depression)

Summary: The care of patients with depression is often challenging for various reasons. Patients may not be willing to reveal their sadness and other negative emotions. Physical symptoms can mask the underlying depression. Patients who are passive, speak softly, and do not bring issues to the forefront are seen as just quiet, introverted people. In addition, many patients are reluctant to accept a mental health referral, preferring to see their problems as medical.

After diagnosis, many depressed patients are managed entirely in primary medical care settings and only referred to a psychiatrist when the medical regimen requires multiple medications, or when the patient does not improve within the first months of treatment. The case of Betty Ann described in this chapter highlights the complexity of clinical depression including diagnosis, course of illness, and treatment. Betty Ann began to experience low mood and isolation as a young grade-school student. Along with these emotional symptoms, she had physical manifestations, particularly gastrointestinal symptoms and headaches. She represented an unusual case of depression, in which physical symptoms were moderate for years, then exploded in a dramatic fashion.

The Pathways Model guided Betty Ann through Levels One and Two, though only small improvements occurred. Just before beginning Pathways Level Three, a marital crisis occurred, her physical symptoms overwhelmed her, and this finally broke down the psychological defences that prevented her progress. Her physical symptoms were initially interpreted as a stroke or heart attack.

Level Three Pathways interventions were begun, specifically antidepressant medication to improve mood and psychotherapy to explore her internal emotional conflicts. The marriage did not survive the crisis. But through intensive work, Betty Ann broke out of her depression and felt hopeful about the present and the future for the first time in her life. With courage and a dedicated treatment team, she emerged from decades of sadness. Her mood, social relationships, and productivity improved. At the termination of her Pathways treatment, Betty realized that maintaining good emotional health would be a lifelong process for her, and that she has the tools and resources to continue her journey.

Keywords: Pathways Model, depression, physical symptoms, conversion disorder, medication, psychotherapy

Healing theme: the mind-body connection

The healing theme of this chapter is the connection between mind and body in a depressed patient. The case of Betty Ann illustrates the combination of physical and emotional symptoms that can occur in complex clinical depression. Her body displayed her emotional conflicts in the form of physical symptoms. These symptoms mimicked more serious, life-threatening illnesses, and her medical team responded with an immediate diagnostic workup and medical intervention. This circular path (unresolved emotional conflicts – physical symptoms – medical testing) leads to further emphasis on the body, instead of on the person's feelings. When there are no concrete, confirmatory medical findings, the professional and the patient become frustrated. Continuation of the cycle becomes embarrassing and frightening for the patient, costly to the healthcare system, and worsens the underlying depression.

The patient is sometimes labelled as psychosomatic – which should lead to better recognition of the underlying depression. However, the frightened confused patient often resists this interpretation. The less experienced medical provider may continue to order further medical testing, reinforcing the cycle once again. Betty found the courage to admit the existence of suffering that had occurred for decades and acknowledged her embarrassment when the sadness manifested itself in a dramatic way. A caring, knowledgeable, highly trained neurologist joined the treatment team that consisted of a psychologist, a behavioral specialist, a general practice physician, and a stress-management expert who worked with Betty Ann in Pathways Level Three. With the support of her team, Betty took important steps towards recovery and achieved considerable healing. Eventually, she achieved a recovery from the depression.

> *"The healing theme of this chapter is the connection between mind and body in a depressed patient. The case of Betty Ann illustrates the combination of physical and emotional symptoms that can occur in complex clinical depression."*

Understanding clinical depression

Depression is one of the most common emotional illnesses worldwide. Beyond personal suffering, the depressed person cannot function at optimal levels, thus affecting personal and often organizational productivity. Depression is a chronic condition in which the person suffers from sadness, loses motivation, tends to be irritable, and feels hopeless. Physical symptoms are part of the diagnostic criteria for depression and accompany the sad mood – mostly fatigue, early morning awakening, not feeling rested after a night's sleep, and changes in appetite, either increased or decreased, and less interest in previously pleasurable activities, including sex. Activities that were once highly anticipated are now forgotten or set aside. The first episode can occur during childhood, the teen years, or any time in adulthood.

Degrees of severity and duration of symptoms vary with each episode. Improvements in mood can occur without treatment, and then a personal loss or disappointment might retrigger another period of depression.

> *"Depression is one of the most common emotional illnesses worldwide. Beyond personal suffering, the depressed person cannot function at optimal levels, thus affecting personal and often organizational productivity."*

Physical symptoms often result from the internalization of emotional symptoms, in this case, depressed mood into one or more bodily systems, such as the cardiovascular, muscular, or gastrointestinal systems. Both patients and medical providers focus on these physical symptoms and often do not consider the mind-body connection, overlooking the patient's very serious emotional distress. Recent research has enlightened the association between depression and inflammation; specifically, that the physical symptoms arise from an underlying inflammatory process, which worsens the depressive state.

There are several subtypes of depression. Dysthymia comprises two years of milder symptoms of sadness and loss of interest. Major depression requires a minimum of two weeks or more of severe sadness and loss of interest and motivation. Some people have "double depression": the first layer is a chronic pattern of mild symptoms, and the second layer involves more severe but intermittent episodes of "major depression". Brief paper and pencil or electronic screeners for depression and anxiety have become part of yearly wellness visits in primary care practices and most medical specialities. These are not sufficient for a final diagnosis, but they are very useful to engage patients in conversation about their mood.

> *"Physical symptoms often result from the internalization of emotional symptoms, in this case, depression into one or more bodily systems, such as the cardiovascular, muscular, or gastrointestinal systems."*

Depression impairs function to varying degrees. Depressed children are often quiet and do not make trouble, but make few friends. Depressed teens may have one or two friends, but are not viewed as social in larger groups. Depressed adult employees do not function to the best of their ability and capacity. They are passed over for promotion because they lack confidence and do not advocate for themselves. In relationships, depressed men and women may seek more dominating partners so they don't have to make decisions.

The risk of suicide must be assessed in every person who is evaluated and treated for depression. The risk increases when the person experiences a crisis, symptoms worsen, or the patient does not benefit from treatment. Hopelessness about the future is a significant danger signal to the provider. Patients may exhibit suicidal gestures, such as hair pulling, cutting, or picking at their skin, among other self-injurious behaviors, instead of overtly mentioning self-harm. The "gestures" are mostly hidden from others and are a source of embarrassment when discovered. Whenever a patient gives a positive response to the question regarding self-harm on the depression questionnaire, it is time for the clinical practitioner to pay attention and immediately address the potential for suicide with the patient.

> *"The risk of suicide must be assessed in every person who is evaluated and treated for depression. The risk increases when the person experiences a crisis, symptoms worsen, or the patient does not benefit from treatment."*

Dramatic physical displays are uncommon in depressed individuals and their appearance will usually result in an emergency room visit and extensive medical workup. An astute clinician may diagnose a functional disorder such as psychogenic movement disorder, psychosomatic illness, or conversion disorder. This terminology is likely to create further defensive reactions from the patient – the message that the symptoms are not backed up by data or physical findings signals to the patient and family that emotional factors are triggering the physical response, and this is not welcome news. The clinician delivering this information needs to be compassionate, but also firm, and must not be derailed into ordering more extensive testing, which the patient will probably request. Sometimes, it can help to emphasize the reality that most long-term conditions are mind-body problems. The message of a behavioral health referral does not mean that the disorder is "in your head" or imaginary. Rather, the problem is a mind-body one, and behavioral and lifestyle changes can often bring relief. Nonetheless, it is important to understand that the connection between the symptoms and the internal emotional conflicts is not accessible to the patient's conscious mind at that time.

Repeated episodes of depression are often simply treated with antidepressant medication. Instead, we propose a lifestyle-oriented Pathways approach to the treatment of depression. Medication may be helpful at any stage of intervention. However, medication should be used as part of a comprehensive treatment plan, including attention to self-care, lifestyle, coping, stress management, and relationship support. Medication should usually not be the first, nor the only, treatment. Referral to a therapist for psychotherapy accompanies the initiation of medical management, but many patients do not accept the referral. Major types of therapy with proven effectiveness are cognitive behavioral therapy (CBT), psychodynamic therapy, and supportive therapy. Lifestyle changes, such as increasing physical activity or improving nutrition, are often recommended as part of a comprehensive regimen, but they also have specific effectiveness for clinical depression.

Introducing Betty Ann

Betty Ann first experienced times of sadness in second grade, some of which lasted one or two weeks. She had trouble staying on task and felt stupid when she got behind in classroom work. Her older sister had attended the same school and had been a top student and a star on the soccer field. Betty Ann was neither of those things; rather, she was a dreamy, beautiful blonde girl who rarely smiled. Teachers yelled at her when she lost concentration, and her peers called her "flaky". Betty Ann frequently told her parents that her stomach hurt, or she had a headache, and she couldn't go to school. They did not often let her stay home since her parents both worked, and they did not have anyone available to come and care for Betty. So she was dropped off at school squinting in the sun due to the headache, feeling sick, and wanting the day to be over.

During her teenage years, Betty Ann had only one close friend, a girl in her class whose parents were divorcing. Sherry was another sad child who worried about the possibility of changing schools, and shuttling between the parents. Betty Ann started worrying about the same issues, sure that both parents would choose her older sister, and she (Betty) would have to live with a relative. Once, during an intense conversation with Sherry, Betty mentioned that she had cut herself. Sherry was disgusted, turned around and went home. Betty was devastated; she ran after Sherry saying: "I didn't mean to say that; I was thinking about a movie that I saw". She continued cutting in secret, fearful that someone would find out, but needing the relief from emotional pain that self-harm can temporarily provide.

Betty Ann was obviously sad, but school counselors blamed the sadness on her physical symptoms. They advised her against going to college since they thought she would not be able to function in higher-level classes, or in that social setting. But surprising many, Betty believed that she might be interested in some of the college classes and that escaping the high-school routines and criticism by other students would help her feel better. She applied to the local college and was accepted. She lived at home with her parents, and worked part time during the semesters and full time during the summers.

Betty Ann met Brandon in her junior year. He was ten years older than Betty, a librarian and teacher at the small local college. He was quiet in social situations unless the topics turned to philosophy or the meaning of life, where he considered himself an expert. Betty thought Brandon was a genius and was flattered that he was interested in her. Brandon did not complain when Betty did not want to go out on a date but preferred to stay in at his apartment and watch TV. They married when Betty graduated from college, and she moved into Brandon's apartment.

As Betty Ann and Brandon became intimate, it became clear to Betty that they were not sexually compatible. Brandon called Betty – "*his* beautiful blonde with the perfect body" and desired sexual intimacy frequently. He enjoyed rougher sex and did not often consider Betty's needs. Betty did not complain but did sometimes decline intimacy because of a headache or upset stomach, which angered Brandon.

Two children, a boy and a girl, were born within five years. Both Betty and Brandon were good parents to the children. They agreed on what constitutes good parenting, what responsibility the kids should have, and how they should be disciplined. When one of the kids complained of a headache and didn't want to go to school, Betty kept the child home or asked her mother to come to babysit, not wanting her children to repeat her own miserable days in grade school. But the couple argued more frequently about money, the cost of Betty's frequent medical appointments, and their incompatibility in the bedroom. Brandon made fun of Betty's part-time job, comparing her work to his much more intellectual profession – now head of the library at the college.

Betty Ann had a part-time job at the local community centre She mostly did computer work, entering information about classes, registrations, and memberships. Parents and their kids were always in the facility and, surprisingly, she enjoyed the enthusiasm around her. She was more comfortable interacting with the kids than with the parents, but nonetheless obtained the necessary information from the parents and completed tasks on time and correctly.

When Betty Ann was thirty-nine, her doctor began to use screening questionnaires in his office. He was shocked at Betty Ann's scores. Her PHQ-9 (depression inventory) score was 18 (indicating severe depression) and her answer to question 9, "Have you ever thought about hurting yourself", was "often". He wanted to refer Betty Ann to a psychiatrist, but she refused. Her explanation was, "I want to see specialists for my headaches, for my digestive problems; anyone would be sad if their stomach hurt all the time". The physician suggested that there was a program called "Pathways" that considered physical and emotional problems. It was not a psychiatric practice, but rather a team of providers specializing in chronic health problems. Betty agreed to try it when the physician told her that Pathways was not exclusively for mental health problems.

The Pathways journey: assessment

With the guidance of a behavioral specialist, Betty rated her level of wellbeing in ten areas in her Pathways Assessment. She rated herself from *one* to *five* in each area, with one indicating very low functioning in an area, and five indicating high levels of wellbeing in that area.

> *"With the guidance of a behavioral specialist, Betty rated her level of wellbeing in ten areas in her Pathways Assessment."*

- Emotional wellbeing
- Cognitive wellbeing
- Physical wellbeing
- Nutritional wellbeing
- Substance use wellbeing
- Sleep wellbeing
- Social/relationship wellbeing
- Spiritual wellbeing
- Illness self-management
- Readiness for change

Emotional wellbeing: Betty acknowledged her sadness and her times of anxiousness, admitting that she worried about her physical symptoms and many other things. She rated herself as a *one* to *two*.

Cognitive wellbeing: Betty rated herself a *one*. "I was always told that I was stupid; I had trouble in school and barely graduated from college. I work a simple job and Brandon takes care of all the finances. Brandon tries to explain financial planning and budgeting to me, but I don't understand it; then sometimes Brandon calls me stupid." The evaluator reminded Betty that she was a college graduate and that only a third of the population holds a college degree. Betty's self-rating changed to a *"reluctant two"*.

Physical wellbeing: Betty rated herself a *four* out of five. She took walks and rode her bicycle at least three times a week. She enjoyed being outside in most weather, resorting to indoor walking during the worst winter months.

Nutritional wellbeing: Betty rated herself a *four*. She paid attention to her weight which did not fluctuate more than one or two pounds; she was careful with high-sugar or high-fat foods, and she checked labels for salt content. Betty did most of the cooking because neither she nor Brandon liked fast food. They both wanted their kids to have healthy nourishing meals.

Substance use wellbeing: She admitted to overusing alcohol several times a month. She and Brandon often watched a movie on weekend nights and drank a six-pack of beer each. She rated herself a *two*. She never used any illegal drugs.

Sleep wellbeing: Betty had little trouble going to sleep because she felt exhausted by the end of the day, but she woke up early and couldn't go back to sleep. She did not feel rested in the morning, and she was tired by late afternoon. She took a nap whenever she had the chance. She rated herself a *two* on sleep.

Social/relationship wellbeing: Betty rated herself a *two* because she felt awkward in social situations. She and Brandon had few friends, mostly people from Brandon's job. They recognized the parents of their children's schoolmates but did not socialize with them. When asked to name her closest friend, Betty Ann stated – "I guess my mother".

Spiritual wellbeing: Betty said that she had lost her faith. She was raised a Lutheran Christian but did not feel a connection to that faith or any other organized religious group. When asked about her spirituality, she replied that she was too dumb to be spiritual and rated herself a *two*.

Illness self-management: With tears in her eyes, Betty rated herself a *one* to *two*. "I often feel sick, and I don't get any help from medication. I don't know what to do to feel better."

Readiness for change: Betty admitted that she appreciated her primary care physician taking her seriously. When he explained the scores on the two screening questionnaires, Betty had mixed feelings: "Am I really that depressed compared to other people?" And "I have felt sad for as long as I can remember". She did not want to see a psychiatrist, but she genuinely wanted to feel better. She did not cut herself anymore, but the thoughts of suicide recurred whenever she was overtired or under time pressure or arguing with Brandon. She rated herself a *three*.

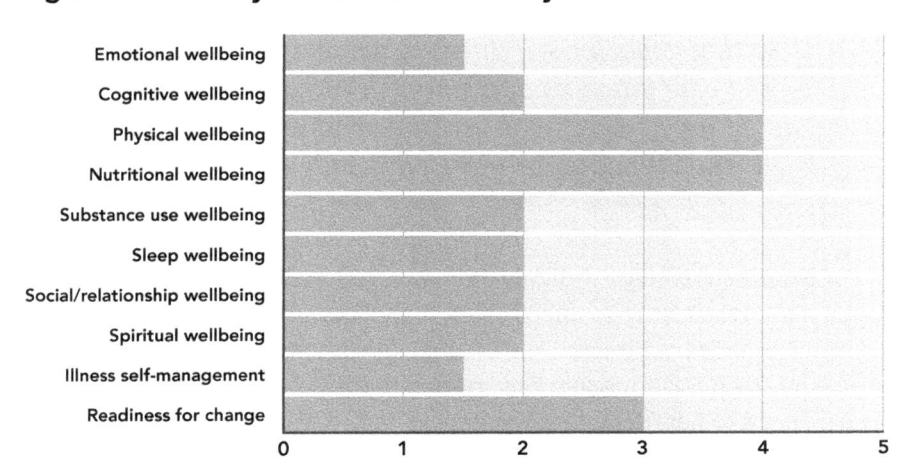

Figure 10.1: Betty Ann's initial Pathways self-assessment

Category	Rating
Emotional wellbeing	1.5
Cognitive wellbeing	2
Physical wellbeing	4
Nutritional wellbeing	4
Substance use wellbeing	2
Sleep wellbeing	0
Social/relationship wellbeing	0
Spiritual wellbeing	0
Illness self-management	1.5
Readiness for change	3

Pathways treatment

Level One goals

Level One in the Pathways Model involves setting goals for self-directed changes, including self-care practices and simple lifestyle changes. Betty's Level One goals were to improve nutrition and be more physically active. The behavioral specialist was surprised by these goals since Betty rated herself *four* to *five* on both of these assessment areas. However, he believed it was important to support her in whatever goals she set, while suggesting other Level One interventions that might also be helpful. Betty consistently went back in conversation to her physical symptoms, which gave the provider the idea to recommend slow, paced breathing. He provided Betty with evidence that breathing is beneficial in reducing headaches and improving sleep. He instructed her to practice the breathing exercise for five minutes several times a day and ten minutes before bedtime (Appendix A provides instructions for mindful, paced diaphragmatic breathing). He also recommended discontinuing naps, a basic guideline of sleep medicine.

> *"Level One in the Pathways Model involves setting goals for self-directed changes, including self-care practices and simple lifestyle changes. Betty's Level One goals were to improve nutrition and be more physically active."*

One of Betty's co-workers regularly attended the local non-denominational church and invited Betty to attend the weekly discussion groups. Both times that Betty attended the topics were on dealing with guilt and remorse. Betty became so anxious during the conversation that she had to leave the room. She explained to her friend that she did not feel well; then reported at her next Pathways appointment that she could not go back. "There were actions in my past that I regret but cannot talk about at this time."

Level One progress

Increased movement and improved nutrition were far from top priorities in the opinion of the Pathways team, but Betty took these goals seriously. She started lifting weights several times a week and adopted a consistent schedule for walking. She felt stronger and felt a sense of accomplishment. For the nutrition goal, she added one additional fruit or vegetable each day.

Betty had difficulty with the breath training. She had difficulty keeping up the paced breathing for more than a few minutes at a time because her mind would not settle. Regarding sleep, Betty decreased the length of her naps but did not eliminate them. She noticed that she was sleeping about thirty minutes longer and feeling slightly more rested in the morning.

Level Two goals

Level Two goals continue to emphasize self-care but draw more extensively on external assistance and community-based resources. Betty Ann was introduced to the progressive muscle relaxation exercise and followed the instructor as he demonstrated the cycle of tensing the muscles, holding the tension while observing the sensations of tension, and then relaxing (tense – hold – relax). Then they practiced together. (Appendix A includes instructions for progressive muscle relaxation and Appendix B includes a web link for a YouTube video on progressive muscle relaxation.) Daily practice was recommended, to include brief, slow breathing, followed by progressive muscle relaxation.

Improving communication with others was another Level Two goal. Betty admitted that the communication between herself and Brandon had deteriorated, but she was reluctant to try to improve their marital communication at that time. She was willing to work on being more comfortable talking with her colleagues at work and the parents who were members of the community centre. Betty practiced sample statements to use at work. At first, she felt silly, but then became more comfortable asking simple personal questions: "That's a great coat – where did you get it" or stating facts that could not be contested such as: "This is the coldest morning in the whole week". She used the practice phrases more often and then developed phrases on her own.

Level Two progress

Betty responded well to the progressive muscle relaxation exercise, describing the positive sensations of relaxed muscles. She explained that starting with a few slow breaths, then moving to the tense – hold – relax exercise did not pose the same challenges as doing the breath exercise alone. She experienced a sense of control and said that her mood had improved quite a bit. Betty was also proud of her progress in being able to talk to her co-workers with less awkwardness. She stated that she felt much less depressed and that perhaps this was the best that she could achieve in Pathways. The behavioral specialist re-tested her with the PHQ. Betty's score had only decreased a few points – indicating that she was still clinically depressed. The question on thoughts of suicide had improved from "often" to "sometimes", but was still not a zero. The specialist suggested that no one can predict the total progress that a person will make and recommended that Betty continue to Level Three. At this suggestion, Betty restated her refusal to see a psychiatrist.

> *"Betty responded well to the progressive muscle relaxation exercise, describing the positive sensations of relaxed muscles."*

Three months after the initiation of the Pathways program, an appointment was set up for Betty with the team to consider the Level Three options. Betty Ann arrived on time, but her behavior was dramatically different; she slurred her words and exhibited twitching movements around her mouth.

She reported pain in her chest and right arm. Betty strongly denied recent use of alcohol or drugs. With Betty's permission the emergency medical services were called, and Betty Ann was taken to the nearby medical centre. She was evaluated first by the stroke team and then by the cardiac medical team. No evidence of stroke or heart attack was found. The neurologist performed a brief neurological exam and ordered an EEG which revealed no abnormalities. Brandon had been called. He had cancelled his last class and was more angry than worried about Betty. He remarked: "My wife is having another breakdown and this time she got herself into the emergency room. Our insurance probably won't cover this latest 'million-dollar workup'." Betty cried in a childlike voice: "What is wrong with me? Nobody helps me. My head hurts."

The neurologist took over the case and became the lead doctor for Betty Ann. She was kind but firm. She told both Betty Ann and Brandon that when physical symptoms are obvious but cannot be confirmed by testing, the symptoms may indicate a strong internal emotional conflict. This is called conversion disorder. Both Betty Ann and Brandon were unbelieving and defensive. "What conflict?" asked Brandon. "I am the main person responsible for our financial stability. Yes, Betty works at her little job, and yes Betty is a very good mother, and the kids love her. I don't see any conflict."

The neurologist restated the diagnosis in a different way. She told Brandon and Betty Ann that the conflicts causing physical symptoms are not always conscious and never done on purpose by the person suffering. She met with Betty Ann privately and gave her a Healing Pathways Worksheet to complete about Mind and Body in Chronic Illness (see Appendix C for the Healing Pathways Worksheets). The neurologist directed Betty Ann to show her psychologist that worksheet and discuss it with her. She also recommended that Betty Ann return to the Pathways program and that Brandon stay patient. Her words to Brandon were: "Be grateful that the workup did not reveal an organic problem, such as stroke, which, although easier to diagnose, has serious long-term consequences". The physician resisted ordering more extensive testing but agreed to follow Betty, and made herself available for consultation with the non-medical providers in her Pathways Level Three program.

Level Three goals

Pathways Level Three interventions involve professional medical, psychiatric, psychological, or other services and treatments. Betty

Ann's psychologist reviewed the medical records from the hospital and the electronic notes from the previous Pathways providers. She also discussed the Healing Pathways Worksheet with Betty. She explained that conversion disorder results from emotional desperation; the feelings are very strong but cannot be expressed, so the body demonstrates the emotions in a dramatic way.

Not really expecting an answer, the psychologist asked Betty what the conflict might be. Betty Ann admitted that communication with Brandon was difficult. He was quiet everywhere but during their times of intimacy. He wanted – needed – sex often, and was not happy when Betty Ann said she had a headache or a stomach ache. His criticism of her had become more frequent and more biting over the past several months. The negative comments were never about her parenting but about almost everything else. She didn't contribute to their financial stability, they had no social life, and he wanted friends.

The plan was to work on strategies to improve the sharing of ideas and feelings with Brandon, about a number of topics, but eventually about the differences in their levels of desire and what was pleasurable. The psychologist introduced assertiveness training and guided Betty to practice direct assertive dialogue with Brandon during her therapy sessions. The psychologist doubted whether this communication problem had created the intense internal conflict, but was hopeful that their marriage would improve.

The psychologist suggested that Betty try biofeedback as another Pathways Level Three activity, another method to reduce her stress response. Betty participated in muscle biofeedback and temperature biofeedback training. Muscle biofeedback measured the levels of muscle tension in Betty's face as she practiced relaxation. The muscle tension levels were displayed on a computer screen, increasing Betty's recognition of her tension level. With practice, she improved her ability to reduce muscle tension. Finger temperature biofeedback directly measured the temperature of her fingers, providing her with information about the blood flow to her hands. She learned to use both the biofeedback display and mental imagery to warm her hands. This meant she was regulating her own nervous system and improving blood flow through biofeedback, to warm her fingers.

Betty Ann liked the biofeedback experience and the positive reinforcement from the auditory signal when she successfully relaxed. She understood the connection between the relaxation exercises that she practiced daily and the information from the biofeedback instruments.

> *"Betty Ann liked the biofeedback experience and the positive reinforcement from the auditory signal when she successfully relaxed."*

The physical manifestations of slurred speech and twitching were not constant. There were "episodes" of several days when the symptoms were obvious. The chest pain and arm pain never recurred. Betty's Pathways team encouraged Betty to apply her biofeedback and relaxation skills – including slow breathing, hand-warming, and progressive muscle relaxation – whenever she had physical symptoms. The team brainstormed about her slow progress and queried why Betty was still coming when her progress had been so minimal. They decided to again offer psychotherapy to attempt to first identify and then resolve any emotional conflicts driving her physical symptoms.

Before the first psychotherapy session took place, Betty Ann called to request an emergency appointment and the psychologist met her within two hours. Betty had the most severe symptoms since her first emergency medical evaluation. She was crying and could hardly be understood:

> "Brandon found out! He checked my gas receipts and figured out how far I should be driving and how many miles were on the car. The numbers didn't match. I've been having an affair for two years. I re-met a classmate from high school on the internet. He told me that he had worshipped me, that I was the most beautiful girl he had ever seen. He said he tried to flirt with me, but I paid no attention. He married late and he and his wife had a son. He is divorced now. He is a gentle lover, patient, kind, always concerned about my needs. He never criticizes me like Brandon does. He never calls me stupid. But what I have done is terrible and I deserve to suffer. Brandon already moved out of the bedroom, and he got his suitcase out of the closet."

Betty was encouraged to stay at the clinic so she could regain her composure and then speak to the therapist who would be working with her.

Level Three intervention: psychodynamic therapy, medication, and return to church

Betty Ann told the therapist:

> "I was attracted to Brandon because he said he wanted to take care of me. I was always so sad. I didn't want to be alone. I thought we would be a good fit. He appeared not to be demanding. He worked hard and we were financially stable. We both loved our kids. But as the years went on, I had glimmers that there might be something more for us. Brandon had no goals other than to run the library and teach one or two classes a year. When I felt better, I would suggest going out for an evening and leaving the kids with my mother. Brandon would say no to anything that I wanted to plan. 'You'll be sick', 'you won't be able to do it', or 'we can't afford it.'"

Betty's voice became louder and more shrill:

> "I was doing well at my job – I love that job – it seems to make me feel better. My boss offered me more hours and more responsibility and I was very excited about that. But since I started the twitching, my job hasn't gone as well. They allow me to work from home, but I don't like that. I actually miss the people. If the twitching and slurring get worse, it will scare the little kids and I'll lose my job. That would devastate me and I couldn't survive it."

The therapist explored the history of Betty's depression and the circumstances that may have triggered the first episodes in grade school. It became clear that the headaches and stomach aches accompanied the sadness. Betty stated that her body was trying to protect her from experiencing the sadness so that her parents, her paediatrician, and the teachers would focus on her physical symptoms. Being called stupid, and always compared to her sister, she had little self-confidence and minimal hope for the future. The therapist highlighted the positive decisions that Betty had made, for example going to college and graduating. Betty's marriage to Brandon had started out well. She could depend on him, and he appeared laid back and undemanding. The children were a source of joy for both of them.

Brandon's attitudes and behavior changed over the years. He grew tired of hearing about Betty's physical complaints and the cost of co-pays for doctor's appointments. When she refused intimacy, he became angry and sometimes threatened to leave her. He told her she had a better life than most people. The criticism was hurtful; they both drank a little more and became less communicative. Betty gave into the temptation to meet "him" (her high school classmate), only talking at first, then slowly moving into an intimate relationship.

Marital therapy was recommended, but Brandon refused. He could not understand how the circumstances at home, his nastiness and his demands, could in any way have led to Betty's unfaithfulness. He refused to forgive her actions, stating:

> "She has been lying to me for two years, sneaking off to meet someone else. I have been faithful, never strayed. I cannot stay in this marriage. But Betty is a good mother. We will share custody and I will pay child support."

Betty continued in therapy for another year. Her goals were to adjust to living on her own, eliminate thoughts of suicide, and break out of the decades of depression. She broke it off with her lover because she could not reconcile her pleasure with him with her admitted cheating on Brandon. In her mind, the affair remained connected to the conversion symptoms, which she never wanted to experience again:

> *"Betty continued in therapy for another year. Her goals were to adjust to living on her own, eliminate thoughts of suicide, and break out of the decades of depression."*

> "I want to be an honest person. I know now that I have to respect my body, acknowledge the symptoms, but be more aware of my emotional state. It is best that I live alone; we have joint custody, and I will have my children half the time. I am going back to the church because I want to re-connect with my spiritual side. I felt safe and happy at church when I was a girl. The services were comforting. The minister emphasized God's goodness, never his anger. It gave

me hope. Now I do not have the burden that I was carrying – walking around like a fake person. I always felt that everyone in this group of religious people was being honest, but I was lying."

Level Three progress

The conversion symptoms slowly diminished as Betty spoke about her past, her relationship with Brandon, and the affair. She worked on resolving the guilt associated with the affair and cheating on Brandon. She was able to express her regrets and sense of responsibility for the marital failure. "He did not deserve this version of me," she said. "If I could have communicated my unhappiness, maybe things would have been different. Our attention was always drawn to my physical discomforts."

The conversion symptoms never returned as intensely as the first episode. Her headaches finally abated to once a month at the time of her menstrual cycle. Gastrointestinal discomfort was minor. As the time came to end her meetings with the Pathways team, Betty said, "This sounds strange, but I want to apologize to my body for listening to it in the wrong way; my body was trying to save me from the depths of my depression and perhaps the symptoms saved me from suicide."

The psychologist requested that Betty journal these feelings and offered a final session devoted to Betty's thankfulness for her headaches and gastrointestinal symptoms, as they had been helpful in a unique way, until the façade could no longer be maintained. It was a difficult session, but Betty reported feeling a great sense of relief at the end, as well as feeling very grateful to the Pathways team. She was assured that she could return in the future and that the door would always be open.

Final Pathways assessment

To more clearly assess her progress, Betty Ann completed a final assessment process. She rated herself on the same ten areas as in her initial assessment.

Emotional wellbeing: Betty acknowledged her progress, but also realized that preserving emotional health is a lifelong process. She rated herself as a *three* to *four*. The depression screener was repeated again and Betty's score was eight. She was not symptom-free, but greatly improved from her original score of 18. The suicide question was now answered "never".

Cognitive wellbeing: Betty and the psychologist recalled that Betty had wanted to rate herself as a *one* on cognitive wellbeing.

> "I was always told that I was stupid, and I had trouble in school in certain subjects. But I know that I am not really stupid, but just accepted what others told me. I have understood the theory of the Pathways Model. My boss appreciates my work and has offered me additional hours. No, I am not stupid. My honest rating of my cognitive wellbeing is a *three* to *four*."

Physical wellbeing: The addition of weightlifting and increased walking led to Betty rating herself a *five*.

Nutritional wellbeing: Betty continued to pay attention to her diet and her weight was stable. Betty was very committed to her children's nutrition and continued to prepare most meals at home. She often made double batches and sent a meal home with the kids to share with their dad. She rated herself a *five*.

Substance use wellbeing: Betty had admitted to overusing alcohol several times a month. During her Pathways journey, she realized that feeling slightly inebriated dulled some of the difficult feelings that she experienced when she and Brandon were together. After the separation, she cut back to drinking one or two beers on a weekend, and sometimes none. She rated herself a *four*.

Sleep wellbeing: Betty's sleep improved. She was no longer exhausted and drained at the end of the day. Despite some occasional early morning awakenings, Betty felt rested and more energetic in the morning. She rated herself a *three* to *four*.

Social/relationship wellbeing: Betty's work had given her opportunities to interact with children, teens, and parents who used the YWCA. She still felt most comfortable with the kids, and less so speaking with the parents. Nonetheless, she felt less awkwardness. A friendship had developed with one of her co-workers, and Betty was proud to say that they had gone out for lunch on a weekend when Betty did not have the kids. Betty knew that she had made progress, but she wanted to continue to expand her social network. She rated herself a *three*.

Spiritual wellbeing: During her Pathways treatment, Betty twice tried to attend study groups or discussions related to religious practices, but the experiences were negative. She tried again to go back to services at the Lutheran church, where she did not have to interact. Betty admitted that her spiritual wellbeing still had far to go and rated herself a *two*.

Illness self-management: Betty felt more confident in her ability to identify her physical symptoms, and then look for the connection to her mood. She used breathing, relaxation skills, and mindfulness to manage her (now) occasional headaches and gastrointestinal symptoms. Her self-rating was *four*.

Readiness for change: Betty knew that she had made significant progress during her treatment. She also believed that she needed to continue to make progress, particularly in social connections and spirituality. She saw the Pathways Model as something she could continue to implement long after she stopped meeting with her Pathways team. She no longer had the "horrible" secret, so she was more open to listening to change strategies and felt that she could work towards specific goals. She rated herself a *five*.

Figure 10.2: Betty Ann's final Pathways self-assessment

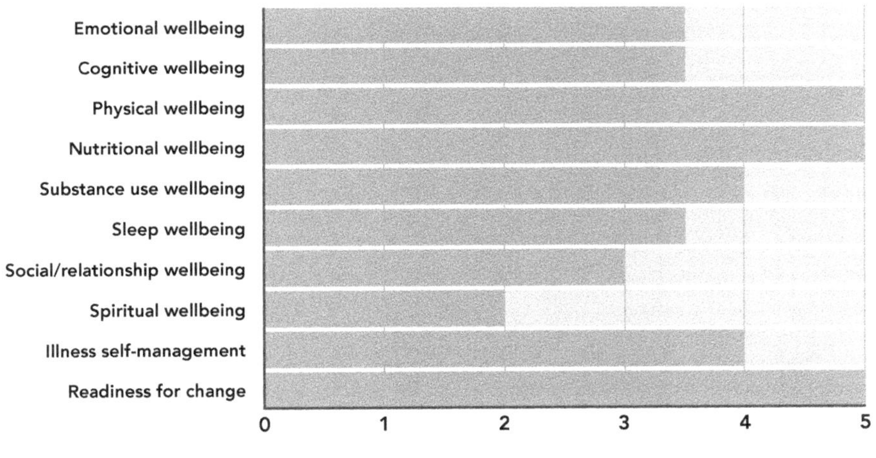

Conclusion

Depression is a common chronic illness that can develop at any time in a person's life. Symptoms range from mild to severe and therefore can affect function to a minor extent or seriously impair performance. Physical symptoms are part of the diagnostic criteria for depression, along with sadness and lack of motivation. The case described in this chapter illustrates how years of sadness and physical symptoms suddenly emerged as a dramatic display of stroke-like symptoms, called conversion disorder. The Pathways team was challenged to first accept the patient's stated goals while realizing that the patient could not set a goal matched to her actual needs at that time. The team continued to offer Level Two interventions and Betty reported feeling more relaxed, more confident, and in control. The conversion symptoms worsened during a marital crisis, leading the patient to draw on Pathways Level Three resources. In-depth psychotherapy, medication, and the expertise of a neurologist helped Betty to resolve the conflict and set a new course for health and wellbeing.

Final message: *The mind and body are interwoven in the development of most long-term conditions. Frequently, physical symptoms preoccupy patients, blinding them to the emotional components of the disorder. A unified mind-body approach drawing on positive self-care practices, lifestyle change, and targeted professional therapies can often aid the patient in dealing with their mind-body problems. This patient initially saw a mental health intervention as not helping her with her headache and stomach problems. Yet, ultimately, Betty Ann used psychotherapy to learn to listen to her body's distress in a new and more helpful way.*

Resources

American Psychological Association (APA). (2019). *Depression treatment for adults*. Available at: www.apa.org/depression-guideline/adults#:~:text=Adults%20generally%20receive%20three%20to,treatment%20of%20depression%20in%20adults (accessed September 2024).

Gordon, J. (2009). *Unstuck: Your guide to the seven-stage journey out of depression*. Penguin Books.

Mayo Clinic. (2022a). *Depression (major depressive disorder)*. Available at: www.mayoclinic.org/diseases-conditions/depression/symptoms-causes/syc-20356007 (accessed September 2024).

Mayo Clinic. (2022b). *Functional neurologic disorder/conversion disorder*. Available at: www.mayoclinic.org/diseases-conditions/conversion-disorder/symptoms-causes/syc-20355197 (accessed September 2024).

National Alliance on Mental Illness (NAMI). (2017). *Depression*. www.nami.org/About-Mental-Illness/Mental-Health-Conditions/Depression

National Institute of Mental Health (NIMH). (2023). *Depression*. Available at: www.nimh.nih.gov/health/topics/depression (accessed September 2024).

Prochaska, J. O., & Prochaska, J. M. (2016). *Changing to Thrive: Using the stages of change to overcome the top threats to your health and happiness*. Hazelden Publishing.

Chapter 11:

Mastering the terror of the unknown (anxiety)

Summary: This chapter explains anxiety disorders in general, and then highlights two types of anxiety disorders: panic disorder and generalized anxiety disorder (GAD). Anxiety is a physiological, cognitive, emotional, and social chronic illness. Emotional and cognitive aspects are interwoven with bodily reactions and behaviors. The case of Eliza traces the emergence of her anxiety from her grade-school experiences through her teenage years and into adulthood, where we pick up her story.

The Pathways Model offers a unique approach to anxiety disorders. Levels One and Two facilitate the person's sense of control over their bodily and emotional reactions to stress and begin to address the distorted perceptions of stressful events. Mental skills, such as positive self-talk, helped Eliza to overcome the terrors of her childhood with a more rational approach to stressful circumstances. Through Pathways, anxiety sufferers learn to anticipate reactions, manage them in the moment, and then work through the negative thoughts and self-defeating behaviors later. Pathways Level Three professional interventions offer in-depth exploration, understanding and eventual resolution of the emotional factors that led to the development of the disorder.

Keywords: anxiety disorders, Pathways treatment, mastering fear, lifestyle, paced slow breathing, sleep hygiene, activity, psychotherapy

Healing theme: years of sadness and the birth of hope

Anxiety is a chronic biological and emotional condition of varying intensity and fluctuating frequency. Fear is the underlying concept that the reader needs to grasp in order to understand anxiety disorders. The fear can originate from one object, such as the fear of snakes, or it can be diffuse or generalized. The fear can occur briefly for a few minutes, or can be the result of previous trauma and take over the person's life. In Eliza's case, fear was instilled in her mind during her developmental years. She was the target of her father's drunken rages. There was constant criticism at home, which prevented her from growing a healthy self-confidence, resulting in her feeling afraid and powerless. Her bodily reactions were an escape; leaving her father's presence to hide in the bathroom became a survival reaction.

Eliza began the healing process by learning to slow her breathing, a seemingly simple task, which gave her the beginnings of a sense of control. Next, more complex physiological training took place. She acquired the ability to relax muscles, increase heart rate variability, and calm her digestive system. Eliza also learned cognitive skills to decrease the effects of harsh or even mild criticism and to assert herself appropriately. The most intense stage of healing was the understanding of the root causes of the anxiety and its effects on her physical health in addition to her emotional distress. During psychotherapy, she relived the terrors of childhood and eventually came to understand that she is a worthwhile person. Her tendencies to blame herself or to retreat from conflicts decreased, and she resolved the hurts of the past.

> *"Fear is the underlying concept that the reader needs to grasp in order to understand anxiety disorders. The fear can originate from one object, such as the fear of snakes, or it can be diffuse or generalized."*

Understanding anxiety disorders

Anxiety is a very common experience throughout the lifespan. Feeling apprehensive and uncertain about new situations, worrying about the reactions of others, or questioning one's ability to perform a task correctly are not signs of a disorder. Normal adults (without an anxiety disorder) often worry about the passage of time, the future, or the past, particularly during life transitions. For example, parents of young children who think their kids are growing up too fast may say: "I am missing being with them because I am working a job and I can't get these years back". Middle-aged adults comment, "My parents look older, and they are slowing down. They ask me questions about things that they always knew how to do. I am worried about them." The newly retired sixty-five-year-old states, "I worry about my health; what happens if I get sick and need a nursing home; how can I pay for it?" These thoughts are normal, if they are not constant, overwhelming, debilitating, or interfering with daily tasks. In contrast, when worry is impossible to control, when the person regularly takes a long time to fall asleep because they are too anxious to turn off their mind, or when debilitating physical symptoms accompany the worry, the person's functioning will be affected and we diagnose one of the anxiety disorders.

> *"Anxiety is a very common experience throughout the lifespan. Feeling apprehensive and uncertain about new situations, worrying about the reactions of others, or questioning one's ability to perform a task correctly are not signs of a disorder."*

In the early years of life, children develop certain fears appropriate to the stage of development. These core fears are as follows: fear of confinement, injury and pain, abandonment, losing control, or rejection. As the child grows and experiences some of these frightening situations, the fear can either intensify or can "habituate". When a preschool child realizes that the fearful situation is actually not a danger or when the grade-school child has learned coping strategies, the fear response decreases or "habituates". By the teenage years, most of the core fears have habituated because of repeated exposure without disaster. Teens have also learned that they can get to safety in potentially dangerous situations, such as thunderstorms. Most adults will retain a fear or apprehension of serious injury or death, and this fear can facilitate adults' motivation to stay healthy.

A critical part of a child's normal development is the sense that he or she is protected by parents or caregivers. Attachment to a caregiver gives a child a sense of security and safety, and fear lessens as a result. When the caregiver is not available (either the parent is absent from the home or they are emotionally unavailable), the child does not develop a sense of security and is more likely to be fearful and anxious. Children need to be taught age-appropriate coping skills to reduce the effects of scary events. Repeated exposure to stress with inadequate support from caregivers, lack of effective coping skills, or repeated criticism from authority figures, increases the risk for the development of anxiety disorders.

> *"A critical part of a child's normal development is the sense that he or she is protected by parents or caregivers. Attachment to a caregiver gives a child a sense of security and safety, and fear lessens as a result."*

Theories of anxiety disorders

The basic theories of the development of anxiety disorders comprise learning theory, cognitive therapy, and biological theories. Anxiety reactions are learned from repeated exposure to frightening situations without sufficient coping skills or protection from caregivers (conditioned learning). Social learning occurs when the child observes powerful adults exhibiting signs of fear. Cognitive theory posits that anxiety emerges when the person overestimates danger, sees threats to their survival in every situation or underestimates their ability to cope.

The biological theories emphasize the importance of stress hormones and brain chemistry as explanations for anxiety disorders. To clarify further, when the person is anxious, the stress hormones, such as cortisol and adrenalin, are released in higher-than-normal amounts. Neurochemical processes release either: a) higher levels of substances that strongly react to threats to survival, or b) lower levels of the chemical substances that inhibit overreactions.

It is likely that all three theories (learning, cognitive, and biological) account for the development of anxiety to varying degrees. In some individuals, the distorted thinking pattern contributes the most to that person's anxiety, while in others, biological factors predominate. This distinction becomes important in planning treatment: specifically, whether medication or psychotherapy should be the primary intervention.

Categories of anxiety disorders

There are many types of anxiety disorders. Some are short-lived, such as an intense reaction to a specific situation or object; this is called a phobia. Phobias are a category of anxiety disorders where the person reacts to a specific object or situation with intense anxiety, such as a phobia of heights, enclosed spaces, or certain insects. Social phobia is an anxiety reaction to being around groups of people, having to speak in front of others, or sometimes difficulty even in casual conversations.

Panic disorder is defined as multiple "attacks" of panic. During a panic episode, the person experiences intense fear, in addition to rapid heart rate, difficulty breathing, tingling in the arms and legs, a sense of doom and/or a belief that they are going crazy. Panic is like a lightning bolt: very intense, but brief. In contrast to the phobias, panic attacks can occur without a definite trigger.

Obsessive compulsive disorder (OCD) is characterized by repetitive thoughts (obsessions), which then lead to repeated behaviors (compulsions). The thoughts are not random but are closely held and firmly believed. For example, the obsession that surfaces are dirty or contaminated leads to excessive washing of the self or surfaces. Or the belief that there is danger nearby leads the person to repeatedly check locks on the doors and windows.

Generalized anxiety disorder (GAD) is a type of disorder in which the person worries, is anxious, cannot relax and often exhibits overreactivity. In contrast to the "lightning-bolt" type of anxiety in panic disorder or the specific target of the anxiety of phobias, a person with GAD worries about many different things; they state that they are constantly worrying and nothing seems to go right. They worry about their job, their relationships, what the neighbours think, or their appearance. When questioned about the source of the worry, the person will often respond: "everything" or "too many to list".

Some of the anxiety disorders are related to stress. To understand the importance of stress, the reader should consider the following example. Mild stress is a situation that the majority of people would be able to manage. Most people would be disappointed or angry after being told that they will be reporting to a new supervisor and their hours will change. Most people would be sad and tearful if a close friend decided to move across the country. In contrast, a minority would not be able to adjust to either of those changes. These people become overly worried and anxious because they fear the work change, or because the loss of the friendship creates a fear of being alone, a conviction that no other person can take the place of the close friend. When people cannot *adjust to change*, they have an *adjustment disorder*. When anxiety is the primary emotional reaction, the disorder is labelled adjustment disorder with anxiety. An anxious person may also act or behave differently because they can't cope; then the diagnosis is adjustment disorder with anxiety and behavioral disturbance.

More severe stressors or traumatic stressors can lead to a quick, short-lasting but intense reaction called acute stress disorder. The person will have intrusive thoughts about the event, avoid any reminders, be sad or angry, and will show physiological signs of distress. If the intense reaction continues for longer than a month, then the diagnosis is post-traumatic stress disorder, which is covered in Chapter 12.

Physiological reactions are an integral part of the experience of anxiety and are part of the diagnostic criteria for anxiety disorders. The most common bodily reactions are increased heart rate, rapid breathing, tense muscles, particularly in the neck and face, sweating, cold hands and slower digestion, abdominal pain, and diarrhoea.

> *"Physiological reactions are an integral part of the experience of anxiety and are part of the diagnostic criteria for anxiety disorders."*

The following explanation clarifies the interwoven nature of the cognitive, emotional, and bodily responses in anxiety disorders. Our reactions to stress are part of our heritage of automatic survival reactions; they are hard-wired into the nervous system. A simple example is touching a hot surface and immediately lifting the hand away. The response occurs before we have time to think. If we swear at the hot surface, that is a secondary reaction, a judgment from the higher brain centres; but the arm was lifted out of the way many seconds before. The automatic survival reactions are necessary to keep people safe; the potential for injury results in the person running away or staying to fight. When automatic, intense reactions occur in situations where the actual threat is minimal, that is an overreaction. The person reacted as *if* there was danger, but the stressor was only mild.

In summary, a distorted anxiety reaction occurs when the person perceives the stress as severe or intense or possibly harmful, and the person perceives their ability to cope or manage the situation as low. Perception or appraisal are key words to remember. The person's reaction depends on how they judge the stressor: is it actually threatening or neutral? Or perhaps the situation is a positive stress such as the challenge of a difficult project at work or running in a five-kilometre race.

Sometimes, anxiety can be helpful in making decisions or in taking care of something that has been neglected. The person worries about the noise the car is making and takes the car in for service. Worrying about an elderly aunt who has not been heard from in weeks leads to a decision to go over and check on her. Infrequent back pain becomes constant so the person makes an appointment with the doctor. Taking actions such as these lessens the worry in normal people. In contrast, the person with generalized anxiety disorder hears the doctor's reassurance that physical therapy will be helpful, but continues to worry that there is something more serious going on and the doctor does not want to tell the truth.

Treatment of anxiety disorders

Medication for anxiety disorders helps to control the symptoms of anxiety and can be prescribed by a general practitioner, a psychiatrist, a nurse practitioner, or a psychologist with prescribing privileges. There are many different choices, depending on the severity of symptoms, the need for a rapid response, the patient's tolerance and, of course, the diagnosis. The general categories of anti-anxiety agents are antidepressants, such as specific serotonin reuptake inhibitors (SSRIs), specific norepinephrine uptake inhibitors (SNRIs), tricyclic antidepressants, buspirone, hydroxyzine, beta blockers, and anticonvulsants. See the website at the end of this chapter for additional information on medications.

In contrast to medication, which controls or alleviates the symptoms of anxiety, the goal of psychotherapy is to uncover the actual problem that created or is maintaining the anxiety. The choice of the type of psychotherapy depends on the provider's theory of why the patient has anxiety. Cognitive behavioral therapy (CBT) addresses the distortions in thinking as described above (for example, the belief that the stress is overwhelming, and they are too weak to manage it). Behavioral therapy could be directed to lessening a phobic response that developed after a child had a terrifying experience with an insect bite and as an adult has a phobia of insects. Assertiveness training is a type of behavioral change therapy designed to teach shy, reticent, or fearful people to build self-esteem and eventually behave with more confidence. Many people who suffer from anxiety have been raised to believe that they have little to contribute; they fear saying the wrong thing or hurting others' feelings. They often apologize for legitimate actions or their beliefs, or for the actions of others. Learning appropriate assertiveness skills strengthens communication skills, builds confidence, and minimizes the anxiety associated with social relationships.

> *"In contrast to medication, which controls or alleviates the symptoms of anxiety, the goal of psychotherapy is to uncover the actual problem that created or is maintaining the anxiety."*

Insight-oriented psychotherapy would be appropriate for a teenager who felt insecure at home, believed himself to be less competent than his classmates, and was constantly criticized by his parents. Upon graduating from high school, this young adult may worry about the future. He will physically isolate himself from others, yet spend hours on social media with people from all over the world. Daily habits, such as sleep patterns, can be seriously compromised because of differences in time zones. A person fitting this description may remain at home, may be reluctant to get a driver's licence and may work at low-paying jobs. These young adults are sometimes referred to as "failures to launch".

Other interventions for anxiety disorders are stress management including relaxation, biofeedback, and/or mindfulness meditation. Physical activity is often recommended as a way for an anxious person to relieve muscle tension. Attention to diet, particularly reducing the consumption of caffeine, energy drinks, high-sugar foods, or stimulants is recommended as first-line intervention.

Introducing Eliza

Eliza was her parents' third child. She had an older brother and an older sister. She was at the high percentile of height and weight during development. Her chubby cheeks were praised throughout her toddler and preschool years, and she was encouraged to eat up all her food. In her grade-school years, her larger size drew a different type of attention. She was "fatty" at school, and was criticized for eating too much at home. She developed bouts of abdominal pain and occasionally vomited, which gave her a sense of relief.

There was almost constant tension at home. Her parents argued about money, about the discipline of the kids, and many other things. Although they both worked, the house always seemed to need costly repairs, which their income could not accommodate. Eliza's dad was an alcoholic; sometimes he went to bars, other times he had friends over for poker. An evening with friends sometimes used up a day's pay and ended with loud voices and broken furniture. The kids heard everything and were frightened. They hid in Eliza's room, which was the farthest away from the stairs to the basement where the games were played.

Even on her dad's sober days, emotional abuse of Eliza and her sister was frequent. They were criticized for being dumb, ugly, and useless. Jeff, her brother, was rarely the target of their father's wrath.

Eliza never got into trouble at school and was well liked by her teachers. She had one or two girlfriends who shared her lunch table. She couldn't understand why at home it seemed that she was always doing something wrong. At school, her teachers praised her for her good manners and being inquisitive. She asked questions in class and this was interpreted as interest in the subject, which garnered her more positive comments. At home, whenever she questioned her father, she was slapped for disobedience.

Her brother was often in trouble at school, late with assignments and disrespectful. His teachers tried to instil a sense of responsibility, but there was no follow-up at home. Jeff played football and people commented that he had talent. Their father believed that Jeff had the potential to turn professional. Father and son watched football together and discussed players and tactics. During the football season, the television showed nothing else.

Tragedy struck the family when Eliza was thirteen. Jeff, aged eighteen, was killed in a motor vehicle accident. Her parents were devastated and overwhelmed with grief. Her mother had sympathetic, good friends and joined a grief support group. Eliza's dad became embittered. He often said he was left with two useless daughters who would not play football, could get no college scholarships, and wouldn't know enough to watch games with him. From that point on, no football was allowed on the family room's television.

Dad's emotional abuse intensified after Jeff's death. Dinner times were particularly difficult as Jeff's empty chair reminded their dad that his son was gone. A few beers after work became a six pack. Eliza's stomach twisted and she ate less and less. The only compliment that ever came her way was when her mother commented that her appearance was improving with weight loss. Often, Eliza left the table, saying she was sick. Vomiting felt like relief as she "expelled" her tension and sadness. She got away from her father, but he would then call her disgusting. She felt trapped at home, with no escape. She was terrified that her mother would leave, and she and her sister would remain defenceless against their father. Her parents had several physical altercations, for which Eliza's dad later apologized, but he did not change his behaviors.

Eliza completed high school, but there was no mention at home of college; there was no money. She was encouraged by the school counselor to at least apply and maybe get financial aid. But Eliza wanted her independence from her parents and that would take more money than a part-time job could provide. She had to live at home for two years after high school, working several part-time jobs and saving all the money she could. The atmosphere at home was still toxic. Eliza's anxiety sometimes escalated to the point where she thought she was having a heart attack. She went to the hospital emergency room several times; the physicians completed their assessments of her heart and told her she was having panic attacks and had panic disorder, not a medical condition.

Finally, Eliza found a full-time job at an environmental protection agency, and found an affordable apartment near work. Her responsibilities were to keep track of the employees' hours, do payroll, enter information, and type reports. The scientists came back from the field and gave her data on the water level in the nearby lake, the composition of soil samples, temperatures, and humidity. When the teams returned, they were exhausted, but energized at the same time as they talked among themselves about the importance of their work.

Most of the samples were brought back to the lab for analysis and that data was provided to Eliza. Eventually, she was trained to create probability estimates from the data. She tried to work quickly but made mistakes. The terminology was unfamiliar, and she had not been adequately trained in the complex scientific language. When her boss corrected her work, Eliza was very hard on herself. She worried that she would lose her job and have to move back in with her parents. She often became overwhelmed with anxiety and had to use the bathroom immediately after a meeting with her boss. This was noticed, but no comments were made.

After six months on the job, Eliza began to pay attention to the data; she read every word of the material given to her by the scientists. She was fascinated with this new world of environmental research. But despite the positive aspects of the job, Eliza constantly worried about making mistakes, looking stupid in front of the scientists, and saying the wrong thing when they joked with her. She had panic attacks at least weekly and arrived at work just in time to rush to the bathroom to vomit. Her worries spread from worry about her own work to concerns about the team going out in bad weather. She asked herself, "What if they are out on the lake and there is a storm?" Her mind was full of "what ifs?"

At the end of her first year on the job, Eliza misplaced an important data set. She had saved it into a file and it could not be located. Eliza's boss called her into her office. Eliza was terrified that she would be fired. Her boss was planning to be critical and harsh, but when Eliza entered her office, she was shocked at her pallor. She was shaking and stuttering, apologizing over and over. She called herself stupid and said she would resign. Eliza's boss took a kinder tone. She promised to help Eliza look for the data and assured Eliza that her mistake was not intentional. The boss and Eliza searched the data files together and eventually found the missing data set. It was "hidden" behind a security screen that was not usually available to Eliza. Eliza called in sick for the next two days, since she had severe abdominal pain and was frequently in the bathroom, expelling her tension and hating herself for being stupid and weak.

Eliza's social life consisted of getting together with one or two friends from high school, but mostly she spent time online. She joined several gaming groups on the internet; she called them "her closest friends". Sometimes, they also watched the same movie. It was common to have drinks and snacks during these activities. Her consumption of alcohol grew as she spent more time online. She believed that the alcohol helped her relax and she slept better after a gaming session. She told herself: "People from all over the world are my friends and they like me. Gaming makes me feel connected to others and less alone."

Eliza had kept in touch with the counselor at her high school and visited her at least monthly. The counselor was appalled when Eliza had a near panic attack in her office while she was describing her "terrible" mistakes and the fear that she would lose her job. The counselor reminded Eliza that she had been on the job only a year and could not be expected to have mastered all the scientific terminology. Nonetheless, the counselor realized that these reactions were not normal worries and that Eliza needed help to control her anxiety. She recommended a program called Pathways.

> *"Eliza's first contact with the Pathways central scheduling office was very tentative; she spoke so softly that the intake person had to ask her to repeat her name and phone number."*

Eliza's first contact with the Pathways central scheduling office was very tentative; she spoke so softly that the intake person had to ask her to repeat her name and phone number. When asked what kind of help she was seeking, Eliza blurted out, "I'm going to lose my job". The first appointment was set up, but Eliza did not keep it. She called back a second time and was told that she needed to keep this appointment or she would not be allowed to reschedule again. On the day of the appointment, Eliza had called in sick to work because of abdominal pain. She arrived at the Pathways Center late. The intake person almost suggested a reschedule, but one look at this frightened, pale woman holding her stomach changed her mind. She welcomed Eliza and offered her a cup of tea.

The Pathways journey: assessment

Eliza was encouraged to rate her wellbeing and lifestyle in the ten areas listed below, on a five-point scale. A score of one indicates very low wellbeing in an area, and a score of five indicates very high health status in this area. The intake worker anticipated that the personal assessment might be anxiety provoking for Eliza, so she emphasized that the process could be divided into two sessions. The approach was without judgment and instead facilitated honest responses; if one topic was too difficult, they went on to the next area.

- Emotional wellbeing
- Cognitive wellbeing
- Physical wellbeing
- Nutritional wellbeing
- Substance use wellbeing
- Sleep wellbeing
- Social/relationship wellbeing
- Spiritual wellbeing

Chapter 11: Mastering the terror of the unknown (anxiety)

- Illness self-management
- Readiness for change

Emotional wellbeing: Eliza recognized that her anxiety was high and she was overreactive; sometimes she could not function because she was so anxious. She rated herself a *one*.

Cognitive wellbeing: Eliza had never been to college but had achieved excellent grades in high school. She caught on quickly at her job, but often felt dumb around the scientists in the agency. Her self-rating was a *two*.

Physical wellbeing: Eliza was generally in good health. She continued to experience gastrointestinal symptoms, abdominal pain, and nausea. She had been diagnosed with IBS – irritable bowel syndrome. When she had panic attacks she felt like she was dying, but she acknowledged, after multiple trips to the emergency room, that her heart and lungs were healthy. She rated herself a *two* to *three*.

Nutritional wellbeing: Eliza's diet was limited by her intolerance for many foods and her fear of getting sick. Her consumption of fruits and vegetables was low; her caffeine consumption was four or five cups of coffee a day. She rated herself a *three*.

Substance use wellbeing: Eliza hesitated at this question. She had experienced the horrors of a home where alcohol permeated the family and did not want to repeat those behaviors. However, she drank continuously while gaming. When her anxiety became overwhelming, she admitted to drinking until she felt the anxiousness ebbing. However, she believed that her drinking was not hurting anyone since she lived alone. She rated herself a *four*.

Sleep wellbeing: Eliza had trouble going to sleep (onset insomnia). She worried about her job performance that day, about the next day and the future. It took her more than an hour to fall asleep. When she had been drinking, she fell asleep more quickly but woke up several times during the night. She worried about not sleeping enough to be able to do her job. Her self-rating was a *three*.

Social/relationship wellbeing: Eliza rarely saw her father or her sister; her mother called often, mostly to complain about her husband. She got along well with her co-workers. She had two close friends. She did not date. Her internet friends were the most important part of her social life. She rated herself a *four*.

Spiritual wellbeing: Eliza had not been raised in a religious or spiritual family. She had been baptized because of her grandparent's wishes, but she did not consider herself religious or spiritual. She rated herself a *two*.

Illness self-management: Eliza was very critical of herself in this category. She stated: "I have had GI symptoms since I was a child and since I still have symptoms, I obviously am terrible at managing my illness. My rating is a *one*."

Readiness for change: The most important part of Eliza's life was her job. The atmosphere was friendly and professional, and the work was interesting. However, as her anxiety worsened, she was terrified that she would make more mistakes and get fired. She stated: "I have to change to save my job and I will do what I need to do". She rated herself a *four*.

Figure 11.1: Eliza's initial Pathways self-assessment

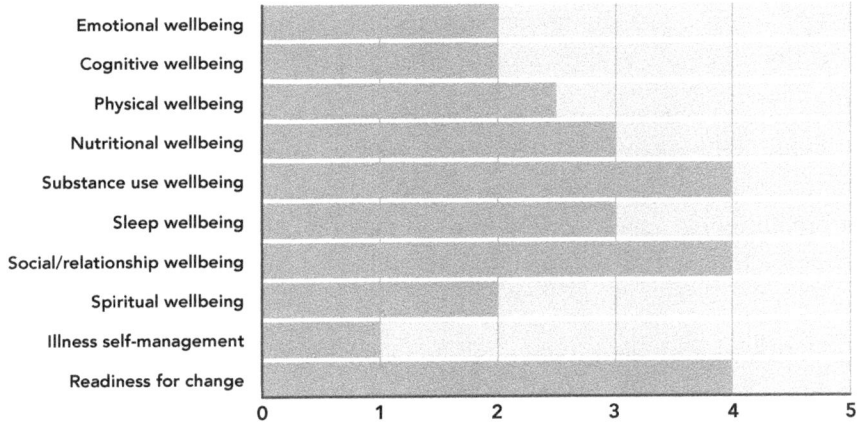

Category	Rating
Emotional wellbeing	2
Cognitive wellbeing	2
Physical wellbeing	2.5
Nutritional wellbeing	3
Substance use wellbeing	4
Sleep wellbeing	3
Social/relationship wellbeing	4
Spiritual wellbeing	2
Illness self-management	1
Readiness for change	4

Pathways treatment
Level One goals
Following her self-assessment, identifying areas of strength and concern in her overall lifestyle, Eliza began to set goals for her Pathways treatment program. Pathways Level One involves setting goals for self-directed

changes, including self-care practices and simple lifestyle changes. After discussion, Eliza adopted the following Level One interventions: slow-paced breathing, decreased caffeine intake, improved sleep hygiene, and increased physical activity.

> *"Following her self-assessment, identifying areas of strength and concern in her overall lifestyle, Eliza began to set goals for her Pathways treatment program. Pathways Level One involves setting goals for self-directed changes, including self-care practices and simple lifestyle changes."*

Slow-paced breathing with the therapist went well and Eliza reported feeling calmer. But practicing on her own was difficult because of intruding thoughts, rumination, and worry. Phone apps with audio instructions and video were recommended, and these helped Eliza stay focused long enough to notice that she felt not only calmer but more in control. See Appendix B for lists of apps, videos, and other resources.

Eliza's Pathways team considered improvement in sleep to be critical. Eliza was instructed to turn off devices and screens at least thirty minutes before bedtime. She was guided to use calming music, practice her breathing exercises, and listen to sounds that she found relaxing. She chose the sounds of rain and wind, which were soothing for her. The onset insomnia slowly improved.

Eliza's Pathways therapist also recommended a decrease in caffeine consumption. When Eliza's sleep improved, she was also able to reduce her five cups of coffee to three. Before Pathways, Eliza's physical activity had been erratic; she took walks once or twice a week, but these were casual and not aerobic. The exercise physiologist recommended that Eliza increase her pace first, then increase distances. Eliza enjoyed being outside and accepted the recommendation to walk twenty to thirty minutes five days a week.

Level Two goals

Level Two in the Pathways program involves acquiring new coping skills and drawing on educational materials and community resources. The interventions selected by Eliza in Level Two were progressive muscle relaxation, strengthening exercises, yoga, and adult coloring.

Progressive muscle relaxation (slow tensing and relaxing of muscle groups, paying attention to the difference in sensations between tensing and relaxation) was reported to be very helpful. Eliza used the exercise multiple times a day and said that she could release tension at home and sometimes at work. After practicing progressive muscle relaxation, she was able to practice slow-paced breathing on her own without the phone apps.

> *"The interventions selected by Eliza in Level Two were progressive muscle relaxation, strengthening exercises, yoga, and adult coloring."*

For strengthening, she was instructed to carry weights while walking, beginning with two pounds, and increasing from there. Eliza reported feeling stronger since she had begun regular walking, and also stated that her mood seemed improved.

Eliza began yoga classes, but dropped out because she found concentration and focus very difficult to achieve. She found a drumming class and reported, laughingly, that she loved banging the drums and felt pleasantly tired after class. The behavioral specialist then introduced adult coloring for Eliza as a way to improve focus and concentration. Attending to the coloring task usually allows a person to disconnect from worries and anxieties: "Take your time choosing the color that you want to use, enjoy the different hues and tones as the picture comes to life. Check the effects of a coloring session on your breath rate and muscle tension. It should have a calming effect on your mind and your body. Certain types of pictures may even have a spiritual connection."

To everyone's surprise, Eliza returned two weeks later with the colored pencils and the coloring books in a plastic bag. She was angry: "I've been staying within the lines my whole life, terrified to make mistakes, scared of my father and his rage, always trying to be the good girl. I will not do this exercise." The therapist initially reaffirmed the benefits of art therapy, mis-interpreting the import of Eliza's words. Eliza again refused, saying with wry humour: "If I'm going to do art therapy, I want to throw paint at a canvas and get my hands dirty". The behavioral specialist found an adult pottery class where students worked with clay and "got dirty". Eliza enjoyed getting her hands into the clay, the feel of it, and then forming something from raw materials. Rethinking Eliza's initial reaction, the therapist suggested that Eliza could use this rebellion as a mantra. "I don't have to stay within the lines. I can throw clay; I can color outside the lines. I do not have to always feel anxious."

Level Three goals

Level Three interventions involve professional medical, psychiatric, psychological, pastoral counseling, or other services and treatments. The Level Three interventions selected by Eliza were medication, computerized biofeedback, cognitive behavioral therapy, and insight-oriented psychotherapy.

Eliza's anxiety was still interfering with her functioning at work. She worried less than before Pathways but was still overly anxious and tense. She had once voiced her worries about the scientists going out in a storm and they looked at her in a strange way, then laughed because they believed she was joking. Eliza was embarrassed, but fortunately, read the cues and acted as if she enjoyed the joke. The panic attacks were also less frequent. She no longer went to the emergency room with panic symptoms, but the few minutes of the attack were still frightening, and she felt helpless and out of control.

> *"The Level Three interventions selected by Eliza were medication, computerized biofeedback, cognitive behavioral therapy, and insight-oriented psychotherapy."*

Eliza consulted with a nurse practitioner to discuss medication. The SSRI escitalopram was prescribed to be taken daily, and hydroxyzine was to be taken as needed at night. Instructions for both medications included the necessity of reducing alcohol consumption, preferably to zero. Eliza tolerated the medication well, reporting no side effects. By the end of the first month, she noticed a reduction in anxiety and her mood improved as well. She used the hydroxyzine less and less frequently because the relaxation exercises helped her get to sleep quickly. She was honest about her drinking, reporting that she was gradually cutting back on her consumption while she was gaming and had stopped using alcohol as a sleep aid.

The Pathways psychologist worked with Eliza to build assertiveness skills to be used at work. It was pointed out that the previous person in the position had a college science degree. The most basic level of assertiveness is learning to make statements about one's own likes and dislikes. The provider told Eliza to state, "I like warm weather" and "My favourite dessert is chocolate cake". Later statements to be used with her boss were introduced and practiced: "This project took me longer than I planned, but I completed it" and "I made a mistake because I wasn't familiar with the software". This was very difficult work for Eliza; she repeated that she could never say these things to her boss or she would get fired. The role-playing continued with modified statements. First, the psychologist was a *kind boss*, then a *boss under pressure*, then a *critical boss*. Finally, Eliza breathed slowly before getting the words out; she learned to take responsibility but not blame herself for lack of knowledge of a task for which she had not been trained.

> *"As instructed by the biofeedback therapist, Eliza slowed her breath as she was used to doing and watched the computer screen, which 'proved' that she had made progress."*

Eliza was introduced to the computerized biofeedback system, which could measure her muscle tension, hand temperature, breath rate, and heart rate simultaneously. The last two indices were combined into heart rate variability (HRV). These sessions were designed by the professional biofeedback therapist. Eliza was apprehensive, but very curious and voiced fascination with seeing the tracings on the computer screen. She had already learned to slow her breathing and had felt the relaxation response in her muscles. As instructed by the biofeedback therapist, Eliza slowed her breath as she was used to doing and watched the computer screen, which "proved" that she had made progress. She was able to relax her tense muscles, warm her hands and increase HRV. The biofeedback sessions had a significant impact on Eliza's sense of empowerment. She practiced at home with a small hand temperature monitor and an HRV app on her phone.

Eliza was encouraged to be honest about her consumption of alcohol while she was gaming. She tracked the number of drinks consumed for a one-week period. Coming back to the behavioral specialist, Eliza expressed shock at the amount of alcohol she was using during a three-to-four-hour gaming evening. It was so easy to keep refilling her glass or getting another can of seltzer. Agreement was reached to slowly decrease the potency of her drinks by diluting the hard seltzer with plain seltzer and adding lime or lemon.

Cognitive behavioral therapy (CBT) emphasizes misinterpretations of events or conversations as threatening or dangerous. Detailed explanations of the stress response were provided to Eliza with written materials and YouTube videos. Her psychologist provided her with a Healing Pathways Worksheet on Living with Anxiety (see Appendix C), as a homework assignment. The worksheet sections that elicited emotional distress for Eliza became the focus of the therapy sessions. Eliza reacted to mild stress with survival-type reactions. Her perceptions had to change, and CBT provided ways to adjust her appraisals of situations to more realistic views. Over the course of weeks, the therapist taught the techniques of countering negative interpretations of events and decreasing catastrophic thinking until he and Eliza were confident that the changes in perceptions were stable.

The most challenging component of Pathways Level Three was insight-oriented psychotherapy, during which the person recalls the past and works to understand the effects that emotional abuse had on their development and current functioning. Understanding the connection between past life events and spending time in the bathroom and vomiting to escape reality was hard. The psychologist explained that, as a young child, Eliza did not feel secure at home; her mother was supportive but often preoccupied with finances and coping with her husband's temper and volatility. Her father was not kind or loving, and instead frequently told Eliza that she was worthless. Leaving her father's presence provided some sense of safety, and vomiting was a way to relieve tension. Eliza herself had used the word "expel" in describing her vomiting episodes. She gradually learned to rely on her relaxation skills to decrease the feelings of abdominal discomfort and her cognitive skills to substitute rational thinking about a stressful situation in place of vomiting. This was a long and challenging process that eventually reduced the vomiting episodes from frequent to rare.

After three years on the job, her supervisor set up a meeting with Eliza at which the human resources director would also be present. Eliza had a flashback of the old anxiety and catastrophic thinking of believing that she was about to be fired. Instead, her supervisor began by commenting that the scientists had noticed Eliza's interest in the data and reports that she generated. She asked questions and the queries had more depth over time. The supervisor suggested that Eliza attend the local community college and take environmental science. She could be a team member in the future. The human resources director was present to inform Eliza of a salary increase and promotion. Eliza said WOW!, and then was embarrassed. They all laughed, and Eliza expressed her thankfulness. Her boss wanted Eliza to take courses in person; evening classes were preferable, of course, but her boss mentioned that flexi-time would be possible if the only time a class was scheduled was during the day. Eliza reported being stunned by her boss's concern for her and her future. She was determined to do well and so she did. Studying took time away from gaming, but she was willing to make that sacrifice. By the end of Pathways, Eliza had completed four courses in which she got straight As.

Final Pathways assessment

At the end of the Pathways process, Eliza was asked to again rate herself on the ten indices of wellbeing.

Emotional wellbeing: Eliza recognized that her anxiety had improved significantly, but she would have to continue to use the relaxation and mindfulness exercises to remain stable. She had not experienced a panic attack in many months. She rated herself a *four*.

Cognitive wellbeing: Eliza was taking college classes and doing well. She still felt overwhelmed when the scientists discussed details of the microorganisms found in the water, but she knew she could progress beyond that reaction. Her self-rating was *three*.

Chapter 11: Mastering the terror of the unknown (anxiety)

Physical wellbeing: Eliza was in good health, overall. Her gastrointestinal symptoms were greatly improved, although they reoccurred when she felt very anxious. She rated herself *three* to *four*.

Nutritional wellbeing: Eliza's diet was still carefully monitored to avoid gastrointestinal symptoms, but she had expanded her food choices and improved her consumption of fruits and vegetables. Her fear of getting sick during stressful circumstances was greatly reduced. She rated herself a *four*.

Substance use wellbeing: Eliza recalled that she had rated herself a four on substance use at the beginning of Pathways. She now realized that she had been drinking to excess while gaming and she admitted that she had been using alcohol to reduce her anxiety. Because there were still episodes, though rare, of excessive drinking, she rated herself *two* to *three*. She committed to continued monitoring and decreasing alcohol use.

Sleep wellbeing: Eliza's sleep, particularly her insomnia, had improved. She used relaxation and positive self-talk about the previous day at bedtime. She turned off all screens thirty minutes before bed. On the nights when she took a long time to get to sleep or woke up several times, she used her cognitive skills and did not obsess about it. She rated herself a *four*.

Social/relationship wellbeing: Eliza rarely saw her father or her sister. Her mother called often, and Eliza went to see her when she knew her father was not home. She got along well with her co-workers. She had two close friends from high school and had met several men and women at the community college. She did not date. Her gaming friends were still an important part of her life, but she now realized that those friends could not substitute for live, in-person interactions. She rated herself a *four*.

Spiritual wellbeing: Eliza felt connected to a higher power when she took her walks. She thought there might be something more, but at this time she rated herself a *three* and felt comfortable with that status.

Illness self-management: Eliza was proud of her progress in managing her anxiety and her gastrointestinal symptoms. She would continue her anti-anxiety medication and keep her regular check-ins with the prescriber. Hydroxyzine was rarely used at bedtime. She rated herself a *four*.

Readiness for change: Eliza looked towards the future with more hope than she had in her entire life. She asked to continue in follow-up with the

Pathways team and suggested three-month check-ins. She did not want to relapse or regress in either emotional or physical symptoms. This was agreed to, and she rated herself a *four*.

Figure 11.2: Eliza's final Pathways self-assessment

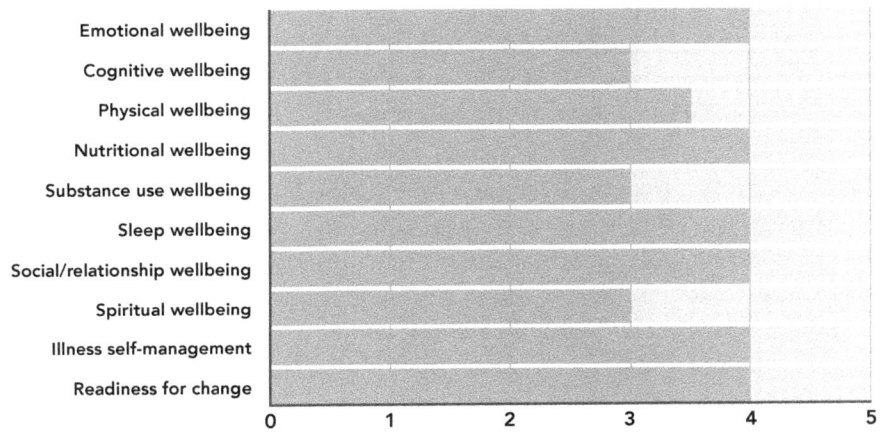

Category	Rating
Emotional wellbeing	4
Cognitive wellbeing	3.5
Physical wellbeing	4
Nutritional wellbeing	4
Substance use wellbeing	3.5
Sleep wellbeing	4
Social/relationship wellbeing	4
Spiritual wellbeing	3.5
Illness self-management	4
Readiness for change	4

> *"The symptoms of anxiety are interwoven through the body, the mind, and the spirit, as must be the interventions."*

Conclusion

In people with severe anxiety, setting and keeping the first appointment may be a large hurdle to overcome. It is important for the intake workers to acknowledge the difficulty and the fear that the person is experiencing and to be patient and kind. The initial assessments may create additional anxiety, so support and encouragement must sometimes precede completing the assessments. No judgment must be the first principle in the evaluation of any person with an anxiety disorder. The second principle is that the healing of the body must accompany the healing of the mind. The symptoms of anxiety are interwoven through the body, the mind, and the spirit, as must be the interventions. The patient must not be overwhelmed *by* or *during* the intervention.

In the case of Eliza, training in slow-paced breathing and general relaxation had to precede the introduction of the computerized biofeedback system. The provider had to be sure that the screen would validate her efforts and not present challenges perceived as insurmountable. Improved self-esteem and success at physiological control, "proven" by biofeedback, had to precede and thereby smooth the path to in-depth psychotherapy. In cases where the person has suffered years of emotional abuse, all three levels of the Pathways Model are usually necessary to support the healing theme.

> **Final message:** *Anxiety disorders frequently begin in childhood in homes where a child learns to be afraid and does not feel secure. Unjust criticism and emotional abuse thwart the development of self-esteem and confidence. Eliza's anxiety correlated with physical symptoms that, in truth, provided an escape from her father's criticism and the grief over the death of her brother. Due to the multiple manifestations of Eliza's anxiety, the Pathways team anticipated a long recovery process requiring interventions drawn from all three levels of Pathways. Healing was a gradual but steady process resulting in much lower anxiety, fewer bodily symptoms, and improved social functioning.*

Resources

Bourne, E. (2000). *Healing Fear: New approaches to overcoming anxiety*. MJF Books.

Davis, M., Eshleman, R. R., & McKay, M. (2019). *Relaxation and Stress Management Workbook* (7th ed.). New Harbinger Press.

Hanson, R. (2016). *Hardwiring Happiness: The new brain science of contentment, calm, and confidence* (reprint edition). Harmony Books.

Rosmarin, D. H. (2023). *Thriving With Anxiety: Nine tools to make your anxiety work for you*. Harper Horizon.

Useful websites

Anxiety and Depression Association of America. (2023). What are anxiety and depression. www.adaa.org

Association of Behavioral and Cognitive Therapy. (2023). Fact sheets of ABCT. Available at: www.abct.org/fact-sheets/ (accessed September 2024).

Bergquist, S. H. (2016). How stress affects your body. (YouTube). TED-Ed. Available at: www.youtube.com/watch?v = v-t1Z5-oPtU (accessed September 2024).

Davis, B. (2020). Stress response. Billings Clinic. (YouTube). Available at: www.youtube.com/watch?v = oE9DNlpXpaI (accessed September 2024).

Mayo Clinic Health System. (2024), Specialty care made personal. www.mayoclinichealthsystem.org

National Alliance on Mental Illness. (2024). Who we are. Available at: www.nami.org/About-NAMI/Who-We-Are/ (accessed September 2024).

National Center for Complementary and Integrative Health. (2024). Relaxation techniques: What you need to know. Available at: https://nccih.nih.gov/health/relaxation-techniques-what-you-need-to-know (accessed September 2024).

National Health Service, United Kingdom. (2022). Treatment: Generalized anxiety disorder in adults. Available at: www.nhs.uk/mental-health/conditions/generalised-anxiety-disorder/treatment/ (accessed September 2024).

National Institute of Mental Health. (2023). Mental health medications. Available at: www.nimh.nih.gov/health/topics/mental-health-medications (accessed September 2024).

Taylor, M. (2021). Adult coloring book: Seven benefits of coloring. WebMD. www.webmd.com

The Royal Institution. (2017). The science of stress: From psychology to physiology. (YouTube). Available at: www.youtube.com/watch?v = uOzFAzCDr2o (accessed September 2024).

WebMD. (2024). Anxiety and panic disorders guide: Treatment. Available at: www.webmd.com/anxiety-panic/guide-chapter-anxiety-panic-treatment (accessed September 2024).

Chapter 12:

Integrating the past and living fully in the present (trauma/PTSD)

Summary: Post-traumatic stress disorder (PTSD) is a reaction that occurs in some individuals exposed to actual or threatened highly dramatic or potentially dangerous events. The reaction to the trauma can occur relatively quickly after the event, or months or even years later. People affected by the event re-live it over and over; they avoid anything related to the trauma. Emotional distress is manifested by anger, sadness, irritability, or anxiety. PTSD can increase the risk of suicide if the person does not see a way to stop the terrifying "movies" in their mind. Abuse of addictive substances is also a risk if the person tries to "numb" their emotional pain with alcohol or drugs. Functioning as a member of a family, as an employee, or a community member is often seriously compromised in people with PTSD.

Keywords: post-traumatic stress disorder, acute stress disorder, trauma, Pathways Model

Post-traumatic stress disorder: the case of Heston

This chapter describes the application of the Pathways Model to a case of post-traumatic stress disorder (PTSD). Heston served 20 years in the military and was deployed as a helicopter pilot on an aircraft carrier. He witnessed combat-related situations, some resulting in the injury or death of his peers. Frequent psychological support was provided to service men and women returning from deployment or after an engagement in which there were injuries. The support could include group discussions or individual sessions depending on the needs of the soldier. During his career, Heston took advantage of these groups and found them to be helpful.

Heston experienced symptoms of PTSD after he returned home to his wife and children after retirement from the military. He did not sleep well, sometimes awakened in distress with vague memories of a dream, and was impatient with the kids and angry at his wife. Surprisingly, his visits with his widowed mother became triggers for anxiety, irritability, and sometimes anger. In contrast to the regimen of the military, his days were now not structured and time passed slowly. Heston began the Pathways program with little confidence that it would help him. However, Levels One and Two were very beneficial as Heston learned basic skills of relaxation and mindfulness and increased his physical activity. In addition, the routines provided some organization to his days. During Level Two, a chance attendance at a community event provided a gateway to identifying early traumatic experiences that had been buried for decades. Pathways Level Three provided support for the difficult psychological work of Trauma Informed Care. Heston gained an understanding of how the early experiences with his grandmother were connected to visits with his mother. Integration of the past into the present, strengthening personal defences and using all three levels of Pathways eventually resolved the symptoms, allowing Heston to resume a normal life and plan for his future.

Healing theme: retrieving and resolving emotionally charged memories

The healing theme of this chapter is retrieving, realizing, reworking, and resolving emotionally charged memories of the past. Heston, the chapter case study, served in the military and saw combat. When he developed symptoms of PTSD after he retired from the military and returned home, his family and healthcare providers assumed that the memories of war were the cause. However, as detailed in this chapter, it cannot be assumed that the most logical and most apparent cause of PTSD in *similar individuals* is the actual triggering event for this *specific individual*.

Heston demonstrated emotional reactions and behaviors associated with PTSD. He often felt out of control after displaying impatience or frustration without justification. He denied traumatic memories of combat, but the specific trigger for Heston's behaviors was not obvious. Exploring and identifying that triggering event is a necessary component of the treatment of PTSD. In some cases, such as Heston's, a current event serves to trigger a painful traumatic response to a past event. The changes that Heston made in activity, nutrition, and stress management gave him a greater sense of control. But only identification and working through the actual trauma, when it became accessible to his conscious mind, led to resolution.

> *"The healing theme of this chapter is retrieving, realizing, reworking, and resolving emotionally charged memories of the past."*

Understanding post-traumatic stress disorder

Stress challenges people in many ways. The stressful event may take them by surprise, may frighten them, or may feel overwhelming. What is extremely stressful for some may be perceived as exciting or stimulating to others. No matter how the stressor is perceived, people need to be able to cope in order to manage the change in their lives initiated by the stressor. Some psychiatric disorders emerge after stressful events. The extent of the reaction and the type of disorder depends on the type and intensity of the stressor, the person's personality, and their personal history.

A previous chapter defined adjustment disorder as a maladaptive reaction in an individual who is exposed to mild or moderate stress, a situation that most people could manage. In contrast, PTSD is a disorder triggered by trauma; most people would have a strong reaction to these types of events. However, not everyone develops a psychiatric disorder after a trauma. Those with minimal coping skills, little social support, few years of education, and a history of adverse events in childhood are more likely to have PTSD after a traumatic event.

Trauma can come from various sources. The classic examples are combat, being injured at work or in a car accident, or seeing others hurt. Another example is abuse, either emotional, physical, or sexual, particularly to children, but also to people of any age. Restriction of movement, being confined, and abandonment during one's younger years can have long-lasting emotional and physical effects. Threats of violence or severe harm can cause traumatic reactions, even if the threat never becomes a reality. Lastly, experiencing and witnessing violence against another human being can be traumatic to the observer.

Acute stress disorder symptoms appear within a few days of the trauma. Four clusters of symptoms are defined: intrusive recollections, avoidance symptoms, negative changes in thinking and mood, and marked variations in arousal and reactivity. In simple terms, memories while awake and dreams during the night comprise intrusive recollections. The person relives the specifics of the trauma and experiences physiological reactions similar to those experienced during the actual trauma.

The avoidance symptoms are described as distancing oneself from situations or people that remind them of the trauma. The reader may consider this to be a normal reaction. Trauma occurring during combat makes the person reluctant to sign up for another tour of duty. But this logical scenario can and often does spread to situations that "remind" the person of the trauma. A woman who was assaulted in the park while walking alone may stay away from that park. What about other parks in the city? What about grassy areas or tree-lined streets? Unfortunately, the original appropriate defence becomes widespread and seriously limits function. This generalization process can be disabling when the traumatized individual becomes increasingly limited in their everyday actions.

> *"The avoidance symptoms are described as distancing oneself from situations or people that remind them of the trauma."*

In contrast to overreactions to reminders of the trauma, the person may also be less reactive to situations where a reaction is expected or appropriate; they feel numb. They may say that they don't remember any details or may experience amnesia about the entire episode. When asked to recall the event weeks or months after the trauma, the person describes the details in a different way. At times, the trauma is not identified as such at the time that it occurred. The memory is buried, brought into awareness years later by a trigger that is linked to the original trauma in some way.

Other reactions to trauma are negative thinking about the present and the future, sleep disturbances (difficulty falling, staying asleep, or multiple awakenings), irritable behavior, and angry outbursts (with little or no provocation). The person may be hyper-vigilant, on guard, prepared for anything, reacting to minor stimulation with a full-blown startle response. Relaxation is difficult; muscles are tense and sometimes painful.

In contrast to the timing of acute stress disorder in which symptoms appear relatively quickly after the trauma, PTSD symptoms may appear a month after the trauma, but sometimes months or years later. However, the symptoms are very similar to acute stress disorder as described above, but the person often suffers much longer before they come to treatment.

The overall care plan for those with PTSD must include education directed to the person suffering and also to immediate family members and sometimes close friends. People who love the sufferer need to gain an understanding of the strange, exaggerated, or numbed reactions that they observe in the person with PTSD. Psychophysiological self-regulation training gives the person a greater sense of control over their mind, their physiology, and their actions. Treatment must provide training in coping skills, and cognitive restructuring to decrease the automatic negative thinking patterns. Consultation with a prescriber is recommended since the person with PTSD may be helped by antidepressant or anti-anxiety medication and sometimes the temporary use of a sleep aid. The Pathways Model is easily adapted to the care of the person with PTSD, but Level Three is usually necessary to resolve and integrate the traumatic memory.

> *"Psychophysiological self-regulation training gives the person a greater sense of control over their mind, their physiology, and their actions."*

Introducing Heston

Heston and his sister Sheryl were raised in a stable home with both parents. Heston was a happy child; he did well in school and participated in school activities. The family was financially comfortable and there were vacations every summer. The kids were disciplined when they misbehaved, but neither Heston nor his sister ever doubted their parents' love for them.

The home atmosphere changed drastically when Heston's grandmother moved in with the family after her husband died. Heston was five years old, and Sheryl was three. As the months went on, Grandma demonstrated increasingly strange behaviors. She made noises, said inappropriate things, and laughed when there was nothing funny or when she was in her room alone. She seemed to always be looking in the refrigerator or cupboards; she had chocolate on her face or crushed potato chips in her hands. She walked around the house during the night and frequently came into Heston's bedroom, repeating nonsense words and phrases. He awakened, terrified, and went into his parents' room crying. Subsequently, Grandma was locked in her room at night, but Heston could hear the doorknob jiggling and pounding on the door.

One day, when Heston came home from school, Grandma was not there. His mother said that she was in a hospital where she would be taken care of. Heston did not have to be afraid anymore. After that, the household was much calmer, and, gradually, everyone could sleep through the night. Sometimes, Heston woke up thinking that he heard Grandma, but his mother comforted him: "You don't have to worry about Grandma anymore". Several years later, Heston was told that Grandma had died. Heston's mother went to the hospital to get her things. Heston caught sight of a suitcase when his mother returned home, which was put away immediately. He never saw it again after that day.

In high school, Heston was a track and cross-country athlete, excelling in enough meets and competitions to maintain his interest in the sport. In college, he majored in aeronautical engineering and planned to enter the workforce with a commercial airline. However, during his senior year, he was recruited by the United States Navy and began training to be a helicopter pilot.

He served for twenty years in the navy flying helicopters, launched from aircraft carriers. He was a very disciplined and good navy man. On two occasions he sustained injuries, once a broken leg and another time an injury to his foot. Neither injury was considered serious and he returned to service after his recovery. As retirement approached, Heston looked forward to a second career and being a better husband to Charlotte and a more involved father to his four children.

Return to civilian life

When Heston came home to his family, he was happy to be there. Charlotte took two weeks off work, and they took the kids on vacation. He visited friends and reconnected with veterans who had retired before him. While Charlotte was at work and the kids were in school, Heston was glad to have the two dogs, Dandelion and Stealth, for company as he often felt lonely. The dogs were a soothing presence when Heston was in the house alone. He walked them several times a day, in the neighbourhood or in the local park that had a five-mile walking/running path.

Heston also visited his widowed mother who lived alone since his dad died years before. When he returned from visiting his mother, he was more irritable and unpleasant to be around. He commented that his mother seemed mixed up at times or forgetful; their conversations got bogged down in details that his mother tried to recall but couldn't. Heston was dimly aware of an unsettled feeling when he was with his mother and being short-tempered when he got home. Charlotte said that other members of the family also had noticed his mother's forgetfulness, but believed that she was bored and needed more to do. The next time Heston visited his mother, he mentioned her memory lapses in an unkind tone. She started to cry: "I know I'm a little mixed up at times, but I'm fine to live alone". Charlotte and the kids noticed the tension between Heston and his mother when they were together. After one of those visits, Heston's son stated, "Leave Dad alone – he just got back from Grandma's house".

Growing concerns

Charlotte grew more and more worried because she knew Heston was not sleeping well, seemed anxious, and spent too much time alone staring at nothing. She questioned him gently about having *bad memories*. He said that he had worked through the memories of the war during the years in the navy and in the weeks before discharge. The navy provides programs to help soldiers integrate difficult experiences and understand their reactions after a deployment where fellow service people have been seriously injured or died. Then, intense and informative programming was offered in preparation for retirement. Heston had participated in these programs and believed that the pre-retirement sessions were very helpful. Heston attributed his restlessness to his uncertainty about what type of job he wanted to pursue. Charlotte thought there might be another cause of Heston's difficult adjustment to retirement, but she did not know what that might be.

> *"Charlotte grew more and more worried because she knew Heston was not sleeping well, seemed anxious, and spent too much time alone staring at nothing."*

When Charlotte suggested that Heston make an appointment with the Pathways program coordinator, he said that he would first see his general practitioner because maybe there was something physical that needed to be addressed. His general practitioner conducted a complete physical and blood work. When Heston described his life in the military and complained about irritability and non-restorative sleep since his return home, the physician commented that these symptoms were probably due to memories of combat. He prescribed an antidepressant and a sleep medicine. Heston refused to pick up these medicines since he denied depressive symptoms and was concerned about possible future employment as a pilot if he was on any psychiatric medicine.

> *"When Heston described his life in the military and complained about irritability and non-restorative sleep since his return home, the physician commented that these symptoms were probably due to memories of combat."*

Charlotte persisted. She reminded Heston that she, Charlotte, came to Pathways when she had experienced severe anxiety while Heston was deployed. She had complete responsibility for the four children and was working thirty hours a week. She noticed that she couldn't control her worrying. Charlotte was recommended to Pathways by a close friend. Both Charlotte and her friend contacted a health coach, who was part of the Pathways team. They set goals and worked on Levels One and Two. Charlotte's anxiety had improved significantly, and she continued to use the skills that she learned and maintained the lifestyle changes that she had made. Finally, Heston was persuaded to try the Pathways program.

The Pathways journey: assessment

Heston rated himself on each of the ten areas listed below. We recommend that you also rate yourself on the same ten areas, on a five-point Likert-type scale, with *one* indicating very low functioning in an area, and *five* indicating high levels of wellbeing in that area. This self-assessment is further described in Chapter 14, and you may rate yourself on the worksheet included in Chapter 14 or create your own record:

- Emotional wellbeing
- Cognitive wellbeing
- Physical wellbeing
- Nutritional wellbeing
- Substance use wellbeing
- Sleep wellbeing
- Social/relationship wellbeing
- Spiritual wellbeing
- Illness self-management
- Readiness for change

Emotional wellbeing: Heston recognized that he was irritable and anxious and that he felt somehow unsettled; he denied severe depression but admitted to sadness and loneliness. His self-rating was a *two*.

Cognitive wellbeing: He was a college graduate and had just retired from a very demanding job after twenty years in the military. His mental processing was strong. He rated himself a *five*.

Physical wellbeing: Heston was in excellent physical condition when he left the military. He admitted that he was not getting much activity since his retirement. His main exercise was walking the dogs several times a day. He rated himself a *three*.

Nutritional wellbeing: Heston had a good appetite and enjoyed eating. When he was active, he could eat whatever he wanted and stayed physically fit, but since being home, he was snacking more, and his clothes were tighter. He rated himself a *three*.

Substance use wellbeing: He did not smoke and drank moderately. He admitted to drinking during the day when he was home alone. He rated himself a *three*.

Sleep wellbeing: He had been a good sleeper in the navy. "When you are going to fly the next day," he said, "you had better get a good night's sleep." His current sleep, however, was less restorative. It took him an hour or more to fall asleep and he had multiple awakenings. He could not remember any nightmares, but felt vaguely unsettled when he woke up in the morning. He rated himself a *two*.

Social/relationship wellbeing: He had a stable family life with Charlotte and his children. He had reconnected with local friends, some of whom were retired from one of the branches of the service. He and Charlotte had friendships with other couples that Charlotte had maintained while he was gone. He rated himself a *four*.

Spiritual wellbeing: He attended church with Charlotte and the kids as this was important to Charlotte, but he did not feel connected to the church. He rated himself a *three*.

Illness self-management: Heston had no idea how to help himself. The appointment with his general practitioner had not provided any help. The physician had spent most of the appointment telling him how valuable his service was to the country. Heston rated himself a *two*.

Readiness for change: Heston stated that he was somewhat hesitant about joining Pathways because he wasn't sure that it would be helpful. But he committed to at least beginning the program because he wanted to feel better and get on with his life. His rating was *three*.

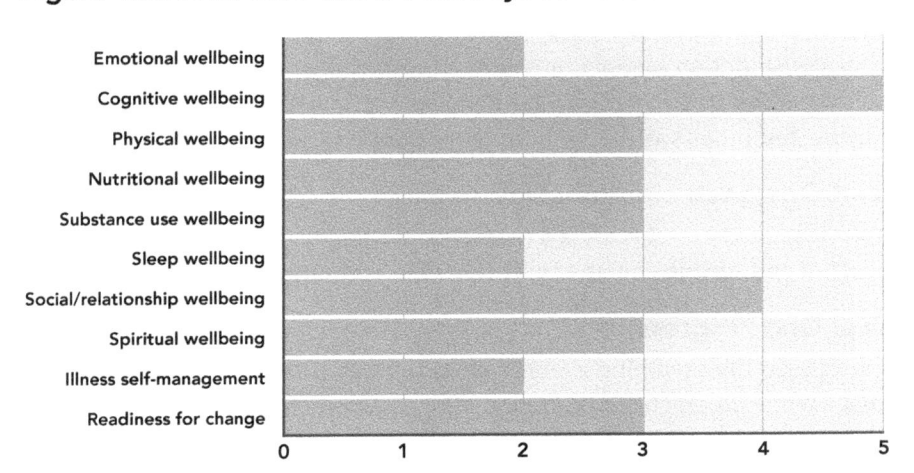

Figure 12.1: Heston's initial Pathways self-assessment

Category	Score
Emotional wellbeing	2
Cognitive wellbeing	5
Physical wellbeing	3
Nutritional wellbeing	3
Substance use wellbeing	3
Sleep wellbeing	2
Social/relationship wellbeing	3
Spiritual wellbeing	3
Illness self-management	2
Readiness for change	3

Pathways treatment

Level One goals

Level One involves setting goals for self-directed changes, including self-care practices and simple lifestyle changes. Heston discussed several Level One goals with the Pathways team and committed himself to breath training, nutritional changes, and journaling.

Level One goal: breathing

Heston worked with a behavioral assistant, who guided him in learning slow-paced breathing using a phone app and YouTube videos (see the appendices for lists of helpful YouTube materials and breathing instructions). He was able to slow his breathing and felt more relaxed while he was doing the exercise. The behavioral assistant observed that his concentration during the task was excellent. But Heston was annoyed; he thought that slow breathing was not the answer to his problems and that it was too simple. He remarked sarcastically: "I was trained to focus one hundred percent. I flew helicopters and landed on aircraft carriers. How do you think I did that if I couldn't concentrate?"

Level One goal: nutrition

Heston committed to two positive nutritional changes: first, to stop all coffee consumption by 3pm, and second, to increase consumption of fruits and vegetables to five per day. He also later committed to cutting back on desserts and other sweets, with no more than one per day.

Level One goal: emotional journaling

Heston agreed to a journaling exercise, consisting of writing down his thoughts and feelings on any topic for fifteen minutes a day.

Level One Progress

Heston used the breathing exercise several times a day and reported feeling calmer while he practiced. He laughingly commented that the dogs seemed to benefit from his slow breathing. As soon as he started the audio from his phone, Dandelion and Stealth came to sit by him and settled in for a time of calm. The change in eating habits was surprisingly easy. He went to the local farmer's market and shopped for fresh fruits and vegetables that the family also enjoyed. Stopping caffeine at 3pm was more difficult, so he slowly backed the last cup of coffee from 6pm by a half-hour a week. He settled on the last cup of coffee at 5pm. The journaling exercise was not successful. Heston found it annoying and reported that nothing useful had emerged from his two weeks of journaling, so he discontinued writing.

Level Two goals

Level Two goals continue to emphasize self-care but draw more extensively on external assistance and community-based resources. Heston reviewed a number of possible Level Two activities, from meditation to relaxation exercises. He committed to three Level Two activities: a) increasing physical activity, b) learning and practicing progressive muscle relaxation, and c) engaging in mindfulness meditation daily. (See the appendices for instructions on these self-regulation techniques.) Heston's physical activity consisted of walking the dogs and playing basketball at the local gym. He recalled his high-school days and his enjoyment of running cross country. He increased his walking to three or four miles every other day and the dogs accompanied him. Dandelion and Stealth were in better shape than they had ever been! The basketball games were originally casual games, but Heston became more competitive and was sometimes aggressive. His teammates reminded him that these were casual games.

> *"Heston reviewed a number of possible Level Two activities, from meditation to relaxation exercises."*

The progressive muscle relaxation exercise consists of tensing a muscle group, holding the tension while sensing the tension, and then relaxing that muscle group while sensing the contrasting sensations of relaxation. Practicing this exercise sequence on various muscles throughout his body gave Heston a greater sense of control over his muscle tension. When he was driving home from his mother's house, he used part of this tense-hold-relax technique and came home less irritated, but still uneasy.

Mindfulness meditation was at first difficult, as Heston realized that his concentration was much worse than when he was flying helicopters. The Pathways team recommended that he read a book by Jon Kabat-Zinn, *Wherever You Go, There You Are*, and also use an educational audio program from Kabat-Zinn, *Mindfulness for Beginners*. Gradually, Heston was able to be in the moment while playing with the dogs, and found that he could also practice being mindfully present while preparing food and eating with the family.

> *"Gradually, Heston was able to be in the moment while playing with the dogs, and found that he could also practice being mindfully present while preparing food and eating with the family."*

Community resources

Heston and Charlotte were advised to attend a local educational series of lectures on mental health sponsored by the local medical centre. Charlotte thought there might be some useful insights into Heston's irritability and restlessness. The first two talks were on anxiety and reactions to stress. Heston recognized some of his behaviors, but was also confident that he had progressed as a result of his Level One and Level Two work. The third talk considered dementia. The speaker described how far science

Chapter 12: Integrating the past and living fully in the present (trauma/PTSD)

had progressed in helping people with mental illness. "In the last century, people with unusual behaviors, people who were severely depressed or misbehaving, were sent to mental hospitals from which there was no escape". Examples were given of problematic behaviors, such as wandering into other people's rooms, speaking in different languages, forgetting to eat, spilling food, crying, and laughing at things that weren't funny. Most of the people admitted to the mental hospitals could only bring one suitcase with them. The goal of this part of the talk was to demonstrate that medicines, therapy, support, and most importantly, understanding the types of illnesses that can cause these behaviors had progressed dramatically in the past decade.

Heston froze in his seat. Vivid images came into his mind of his grandmother, since she had exhibited many of the behaviors mentioned by the speaker. He said to Charlotte: "We have to leave right now". They got into the car and Heston was shaking, trying to clear his head. He told Charlotte: "I think my grandmother went into a mental hospital and never came back home. I have to talk to my mother." Charlotte said, "It's evening, 8pm; your mother may not want company at this time". Heston shouted, "We're going to my mother's, or I'm getting out of the car and walking there. Take me right now!"

Heston's mother was surprised to see Heston and Charlotte arriving without notice. Heston confronted his mother: "Why did you wait so long to get Grandma into the hospital? Sheryl and I were terrified of her; she acted so strangely. You and Dad sacrificed us kids for an old woman who didn't know what was going on." Heston's mother was shocked by these accusations and tried to explain. "She had been a loving mother to me and my siblings. She and my dad sacrificed a lot so that we could have what we needed. We weren't poor, but we weren't rich either. When your dad and I moved my mother into our home, she was okay, but she got worse. We tried to keep her home as long as we could. I couldn't send her away to one of those awful places. We held out until her actions disrupted the whole household. She would never have hurt you kids."

Heston would not accept this explanation. He paced the floor of his mother's house. Suddenly, he blurted out: "Mother, where is the suitcase?" She replied: "Oh, I haven't thought of that in many years. I'll look for it. But now you need to leave as I'm tired and you've upset me." A week later, his mother announced that she had found the suitcase.

Level Three Interventions

Level Three interventions involve professional medical, psychiatric, psychological, or other services and treatments, as necessary. The Pathways team discussed Level Three interventions for Heston since there was no progress in his negative, impatient reactions to his mother and the aftermath of irritability and anger after the visits. After the medical centre lecture and the nighttime visit with Heston's mother, Charlotte called in to the Pathways team and requested an emergency appointment with a psychologist. Due to a last-minute cancellation, the clinic was able to arrange an appointment for the next day.

The therapist met with Heston and Charlotte, reviewed the history of the PTSD symptoms and validated the progress that Heston had already made in Pathways Levels One and Two. He paid very careful attention to the description of Heston's reaction to the lecture on dementia and the confrontation between Heston and his mother. Heston was remorseful about how he had treated his mother, but was adamant that he needed explanations, and he was determined to see the suitcase. The therapist said he would contact Heston's mother to ask permission to come to her home. He (the therapist) and Charlotte would accompany Heston to his mother's house so that the suitcase could be opened.

> *"The Pathways team discussed Level Three interventions for Heston since there was no progress in his negative, impatient reactions to his mother and the aftermath of irritability and anger after the visits."*

A week later, Heston, Charlotte, the therapist and the two dogs came to Heston's mother's home. The suitcase was on the floor of the living room. The lock of the old, battered case was hard to open, but it finally gave way. All held their breath. Inside were the treasures of an old, ill woman who may or may not have understood that she was never coming back home. There were many family pictures with names and dates carefully written on the back. Grandma had drawn hearts with crayons or lipstick on the pictures of her grandchildren. Other objects were a small spade and other gardening tools, and packs of lettuce and carrot seeds. They lifted out a prayer book with bookmarks and notes on certain pages. They saw the shawl and sweater that she always wore, even in the summer, and her gardening hat. The pressed flowers still had a very faint odour. They saw ribbon, some formed into colorful bows. There were love letters from her husband before they married, and more letters from when he was in the service, promising to get back home to her. There were birthday cards, including one from Heston saying: "I want to be a soldier just like Grandpa. I want to float on the ocean in a big boat."

Heston was overcome. The stuff of his nightmares was in plain sight. He was shaking very hard, and Charlotte took both of his hands to comfort him. The therapist spoke in a soft calm voice: "Your grandmother was sick and there were no treatments. Your mother did not realize the effect that her actions had on you kids. Grandma had been a loving, kind person her whole life, and your mother did not want to send her away." Heston blurted out, "Mother, Sherry and I were so scared. I can still see Grandma coming into my room like a scary ghost". Then he went on: "Mother, you are getting mixed up and forgetful. I cannot watch you become Grandma. We have this horrible disease in our family: Grandma, you, then me and my kids will all be sent to mental hospitals." Even as he spoke, he realized he was being irrational. Heston could not stop accusing his mother of letting his grandma frighten him and his sister.

The therapist continued to speak in a calm voice to Heston, reminding him that there had not been a diagnosis for his mother. Medical knowledge has advanced in many areas, including dementia. There are so many therapies and medicines available. The objects in the suitcase and the suitcase itself are relics from a long time ago. They have no power over people currently living. They cannot do harm. Take the positives out of the suitcase. Even though Grandma was so sick, she still loved you and your sister. She planned on putting those seeds in the ground and growing lettuce and carrots, just like she did when she was in her own home. She prayed. She still loved pretty things, like bows and ribbons. She kept the letters from her husband, and it seems that she read them over and over because they are frayed. She kept pictures of all of you and kept the wonderful card from you, wanting to be just like Grandpa. Absorb the positive from the suitcase. She packed it when she was already sick, but what she treasured was family, nature, God, and beauty.

Two hours later, Heston and Charlotte went home, and Heston fell into bed and slept for ten hours with Dandelion and Stealth nearby. In the morning, Charlotte had walked the dogs and given them food and water, but they whined and turned around towards the house during the walk, quickly returning to Heston's side. She left him a note: *Heston, I love you so much; my heart broke for you yesterday. We will get through this together.*

Heston continued all Level One and Two activities. Level Three psychotherapy continued for six months with the therapist who had gone to the house for the opening of the suitcase. Heston's mother attended several sessions with him, and they worked on forgiving each other. They spent time on the Healing Pathways Worksheet designed to help those living with difficult memories (Appendix C). Heston stopped criticizing his mother and instead went to her doctor's appointment with her. The doctor completed a thorough assessment and found very minimal cognitive change. He acknowledged that Heston's mother was at risk, so he prescribed one of the new medications to prevent or delay the onset of dementia. To Heston's delight and his mother's surprise, the doctor recommended physical activity. She was to build up to a regular exercise program, which, according to the doctor, could improve memory and cognitive functioning. Heston promised to walk with his mother at least once a week until she got into a routine. The work with the therapist was very difficult, but finally, Heston reached a place of mental and emotional peace. With Charlotte's input, he was ready to decide on his second career and plan for his future.

> *"Heston continued all Level One and Two activities. Level Three psychotherapy continued for six months with the therapist who had gone to the house for the opening of the suitcase. Heston's mother attended several sessions with him, and they worked on forgiving each other."*

Chapter 12: Integrating the past and living fully in the present (trauma/PTSD)

Final Pathways assessment

Heston was asked to complete his Pathways program assessments, rating himself on the same ten areas as before, on a scale from one to five:

Emotional wellbeing: Heston verbalized his relief that his mood was much more stable and he was calmer. He rated himself a *four*. He acknowledged that some memories came back at times, and he became anxious, but he knew that he had sufficient knowledge and skills to manage the anxiety.

Cognitive wellbeing: He was still confident in his cognitive abilities and looked forward to the challenges in his next career. He rated himself a *five*.

Physical wellbeing: Heston was in excellent physical condition when he left the military. But before Pathways he had limited his exercise to walking his dogs. During Pathways, he increased his physical activity significantly. He was in much better physical condition. He continued to play basketball with his friends, but no longer committed "hard fouls". He rated himself a *five*.

Nutritional wellbeing: Heston's nutrition had improved, and he was proud of how many new (to him) fruits and vegetables he consumed. His coffee intake had gone back to three or four cups a day, but it did not affect his sleep. He rated himself a *four*.

Substance use wellbeing: Heston had reduced his alcohol intake to two or three beers at weekends. He rated himself at *four* to *five*.

Sleep wellbeing: He had been a good sleeper until he came home from the military. Since increasing physical activity and, most importantly, working to resolve the trauma, his sleep had improved significantly. He rated himself a *four*.

Social/relationship wellbeing: Heston had friends and he was re-establishing relationships. Some of his friends had been by his side throughout these difficult months. He rated himself a *four*.

Spiritual wellbeing: He continued to attend services in the local Catholic church with Charlotte and the kids, but Heston did not feel connected to those beliefs. However, he had developed a greater sense of a broader spirituality. He rated himself a *four*.

Illness self-management: Heston rated himself a *five*. He knew what he had to do to maintain his health, and he intended to maintain the healthy lifestyle actions that he had learned through Pathways.

Readiness for change: Heston continued to be open to learning additional relaxation skills and growing his mindfulness skills. He planned to attend the support groups for veterans. He rated himself a *five*.

Figure 12.2: Heston's final Pathways self-assessment

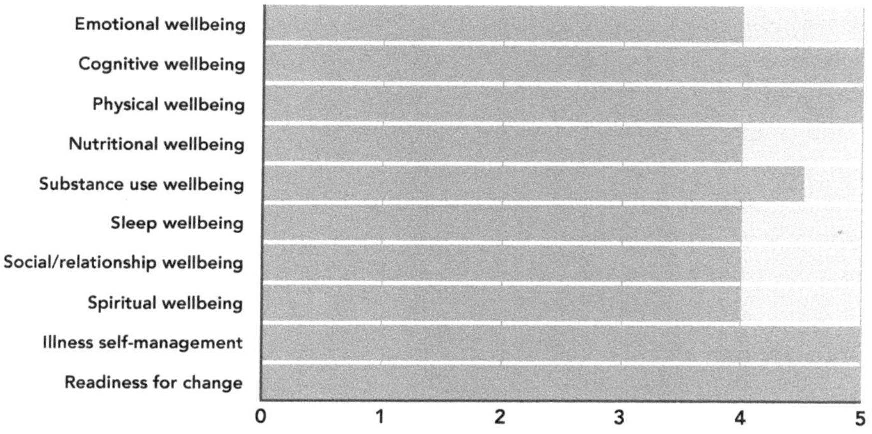

Category	Rating
Emotional wellbeing	4
Cognitive wellbeing	5
Physical wellbeing	5
Nutritional wellbeing	5
Substance use wellbeing	4.5
Sleep wellbeing	5
Social/relationship wellbeing	5
Spiritual wellbeing	4
Illness self-management	5
Readiness for change	5

Conclusion

This chapter provides important background information on how stress of variable intensity can lead to the development of stress-related disorders. Serious stressful events where the person is in danger, sees injuries happening to others, or experiences the threat of injury, present the greatest risk for PTSD. People with PTSD may demonstrate a wide variety of emotional, physiological, and behavioral reactions, but deterioration in daily functioning is common. The case of Heston is unusual in that the expected cause of his PTSD was his war experiences. But as the story developed, it became clear that Heston coped very well with the stressful situations associated with his career as a navy pilot. The trigger for the emergence of his PTSD symptoms was the interaction with his mother, who demonstrated some signs of early onset dementia, and the memories of his grandmother that these present-day interactions triggered. The constant support of Heston's wife and other veterans provided a critical step in understanding and eventually integrating the trauma, and in setting Heston on a path to healing and wellbeing.

> **Final message:** *People may demonstrate symptoms of post-traumatic stress disorder, yet they are often unable to identify the trauma. Patience with the person who is suffering is crucial. It is important for family and friends to recall that the person suffering is actually suffering. Since a sense of loss of control of thoughts and emotions and sometimes actions are often central to PTSD, skill building to support a belief in personal control should be a first-line goal. Pathways Levels One and Two provide this sense of self-efficacy when the person learns mindfulness and relaxation, when they increase their physical activity, and when they take the initiative to shop for food and prepare healthy meals. However, identification and working through the trauma almost always requires a professional such as a clinical psychologist, counselor, or nurse practitioner trained in the care of persons with PTSD.*

Resources

Center for Healthcare Strategies (2024). What is trauma-informed care? www.traumainformedcare.chcs.org

Cleveland Clinic (2024). How to heal from trauma. Available at: https://health.clevelandclinic.org/how-to-heal-from-trauma (accessed September 2024).

Goldstein, E., & Stahl, B. (2015). *MBSR every day. Daily practices from the heart of Mindfulness-Based Stress Reduction*. New Harbinger Publications.

Harvard Health Publishing (2023). Exercise can boost your memory and thinking skills. Available at: www.health.harvard.edu/mind-and-mood/exercise-can-boost-your-memory-and-thinking-skills (accessed September 2024).

Kabat-Zinn, J. (1994). *Wherever You Go, There You Are: Mindfulness meditation in everyday life*. Hyperion.

Kabat-Zinn, J. (2006). *Mindfulness For Beginners: Reclaiming the present moment*. (Audiobook). Sounds True.

National Institute on Aging. (2024). Cognitive health and older adults. Available at: www.nia.nih.gov/health/brain-health/cognitive-health-and-older-adults (accessed September 2024).

Penney, D., & Stastny, P. (2008). *The Lives They Left Behind: Suitcases from a state hospital attic*. Bellevue Literary Press.

The National Child Traumatic Stress Network (n.d.). The National Child Traumatic Stress Network. www.nctsn.org

WebMD (2023). How exercise affects your brain. Available at: www.webmd.com/brain/ss/slideshow-exercise-brain-effects (accessed September 2024).

Section Three:
More guidance on creating and following your personal Pathways

Your personal Pathway program. Now it is your turn. We have provided you with the stories of many individuals struggling with long-term illnesses who have used the Pathways Model to improve the management of their illness and enhance their quality of life. Now we will guide you to complete your own Pathways Assessment and to set goals for the three Pathways Levels.

At each step, we provide worksheets for you to carry out your own assessment and set your own Level One and Level Two self-care and lifestyle goals. Finally, we will discuss how to choose the best Level Three treatments and how to judge the qualifications of available professionals for Level Three treatments.

Remember, in each case, the Pathways Model asks us to be realistic about ourselves. Goals should be chosen because you feel personally ready to make small, initial steps in this goal area. Assessing your readiness for making changes is just as important as choosing goals that are relevant to your illness.

Chapter 13:
Completing your Pathways Assessment

> **Summary:** The Pathways Assessment is a self-assessment tool. Individuals rate their wellbeing in ten areas, from emotional wellbeing to readiness to change. The assessment will help you to identify areas where you have relatively high strengths and wellness, and other areas where you are seriously challenged. It culminates in creating a Pathways Assessment Graph that provides a balanced picture of health strengths and health risks throughout your life, and offers guidance in setting goals at all three levels in the Pathways Model.
>
> **Keywords:** Pathways Assessment, health risks, wellbeing, readiness for change

The Pathways Assessment and the Pathways Assessment Graph

In the following pages, you will be assessing yourself in each of several areas. For each area, you will be establishing a Pathways rating on a scale of one to five. One will designate a lack of strengths or the presence of severe problems in this assessment area, while five will indicate a high level of wellness in this area. At the end of the assessment, an overall

Pathways Assessment Graph will provide a balanced picture of your strengths and risks throughout your life. The ten Pathways Assessment areas are:

- Emotional wellbeing
- Cognitive wellbeing
- Physical wellbeing
- Nutritional wellbeing
- Substance use wellbeing
- Sleep wellbeing
- Social/relationship wellbeing
- Spiritual wellbeing
- Illness self-management
- Readiness for change

Assessment One: Emotional wellbeing

What is your current level of emotional wellbeing?

Remember that the ideal in emotional health is a mixture of positive and negative emotions. Being stuck in negative emotions can undermine your coping in life. However, being able to experience sadness, frustration, or anger when you face a setback or a personal loss is healthy.

On a scale of one to five, mark where you see your current emotional wellbeing. Be honest with where you are right now. And yes, you can mark halfway between two numbers, to rate yourself more precisely.

Figure 13.1: Emotional wellbeing

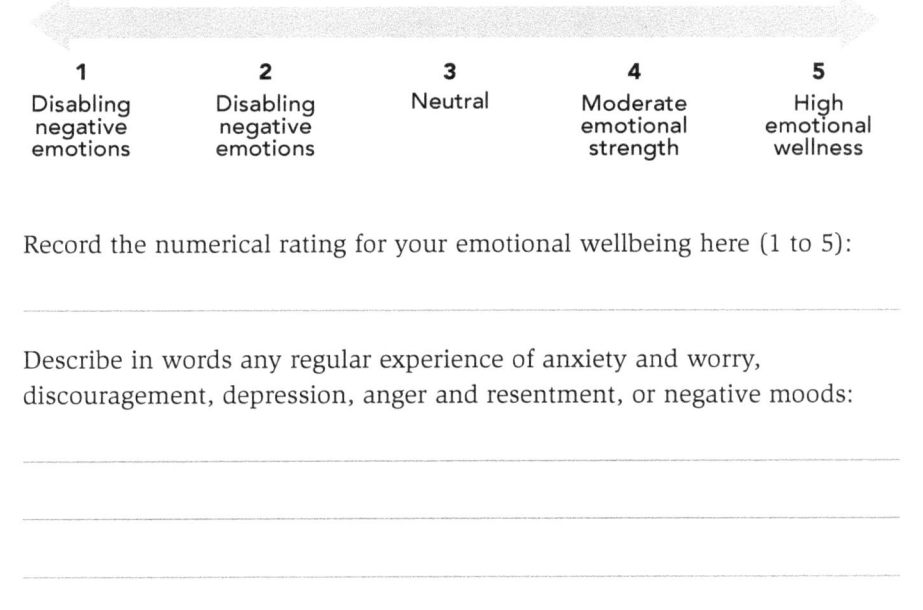

1	2	3	4	5
Disabling negative emotions	Disabling negative emotions	Neutral	Moderate emotional strength	High emotional wellness

Record the numerical rating for your emotional wellbeing here (1 to 5):

_____

Describe in words any regular experience of anxiety and worry, discouragement, depression, anger and resentment, or negative moods:

_____

_____

_____

You may wish to take a free online anxiety or depression rating scale, so you have a measurable starting point for your Pathways program. You can take the same questionnaire later to see any progress.

- The Zung Self-Rating Anxiety Scale is available on many sites online, including: https://psychology-tools.com/test/zung-anxiety-scale (accessed September 2024).

- The Generalized Anxiety Disorder Scale (GAD-7), an online anxiety rating scale, is available on many websites, including: www.mdcalc.com/gad-7-general-anxiety-disorder-7 (accessed September 2024).
- The Patient Health Questionnaire, an online depression rating scale is available on many websites, including: https://patient.info/doctor/patient-health-questionnaire-phq-9 (accessed September 2024).

Take any of these questionnaires now and enter the scores on the following blanks.

Name of test .... Today's date........................

Test score .... Is this score normal, mild, moderate or severe? ....

Name of test .... Today's date........................

Test score .... Is this score normal, mild, moderate or severe? ....

Name of test .... Today's date........................

Test score .... Is this score normal, mild, moderate or severe? ....

Name of test... Today's date........................

Test score .... Is this score normal, mild, moderate or severe? ....

Assessment Two: Cognitive wellbeing

What is your current level of cognitive (mental) wellbeing?

Figure 13.2: Cognitive wellbeing

1	2	3	4	5
Disabling cognitive problems	Mildly disturbed thinking	Neutral	Moderate mental strength	High mental wellness

Record the numerical rating for your cognitive wellbeing here (1 to 5):

Have you noticed any mental difficulties or problems recently? Describe any problems with memory, concentration, mental slowness, fogginess, or disorientation:

Are there times or situations where you find your mental state more of a problem?

Are there any factors, such as food or substance use, that undermine or improve your mental state?

Assessment Three: Physical wellbeing

What is your current level of physical wellbeing?

Figure 13.3: Physical wellbeing

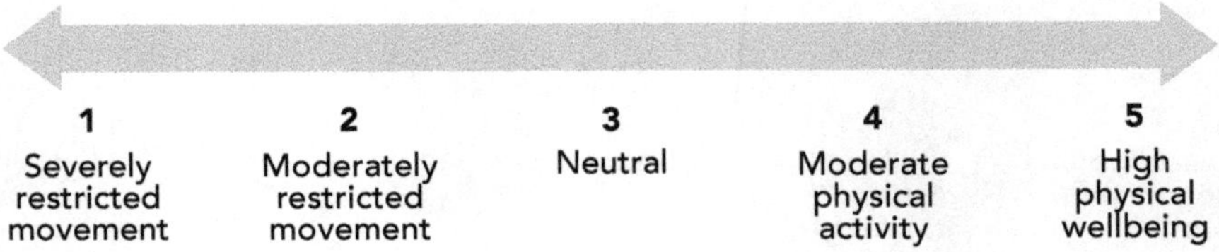

1	2	3	4	5
Severely restricted movement	Moderately restricted movement	Neutral	Moderate physical activity	High physical wellbeing

Record the numerical rating for your physical wellbeing here (1 to 5):
___

List examples of activity or exercise you engage in regularly:
___
___

List factors that prevent you from increasing activity level:
___
___

How ready do you feel to set an activity goal?
___
___

Assessment Four: Nutritional wellbeing

What is your current level of nutritional wellbeing?

Figure 13.4: Nutritional wellbeing

1	2	3	4	5
Severely unhealthy diet	Moderately unhealthy diet	Neutral	Moderately positive nutrition	High nutritional wellbeing

Record the numerical rating for your nutritional wellbeing here (1 to 5):

Describe your current usual nutrition in more detail (mention fast food, take-out food, pre-packaged food, or other negative habits):

Have you made any decisions to introduce special dietary choices, such as gluten free, organic, or vegetarian foods?

Are there any dietary change goals that intrigue or interest you, and how ready do you feel to set a dietary goal?

Chapter 13: Completing your Pathways Assessment

Assessment Five: Substance use wellbeing

What is your current level of substance use wellbeing?

Figure 13.5: Substance use wellbeing

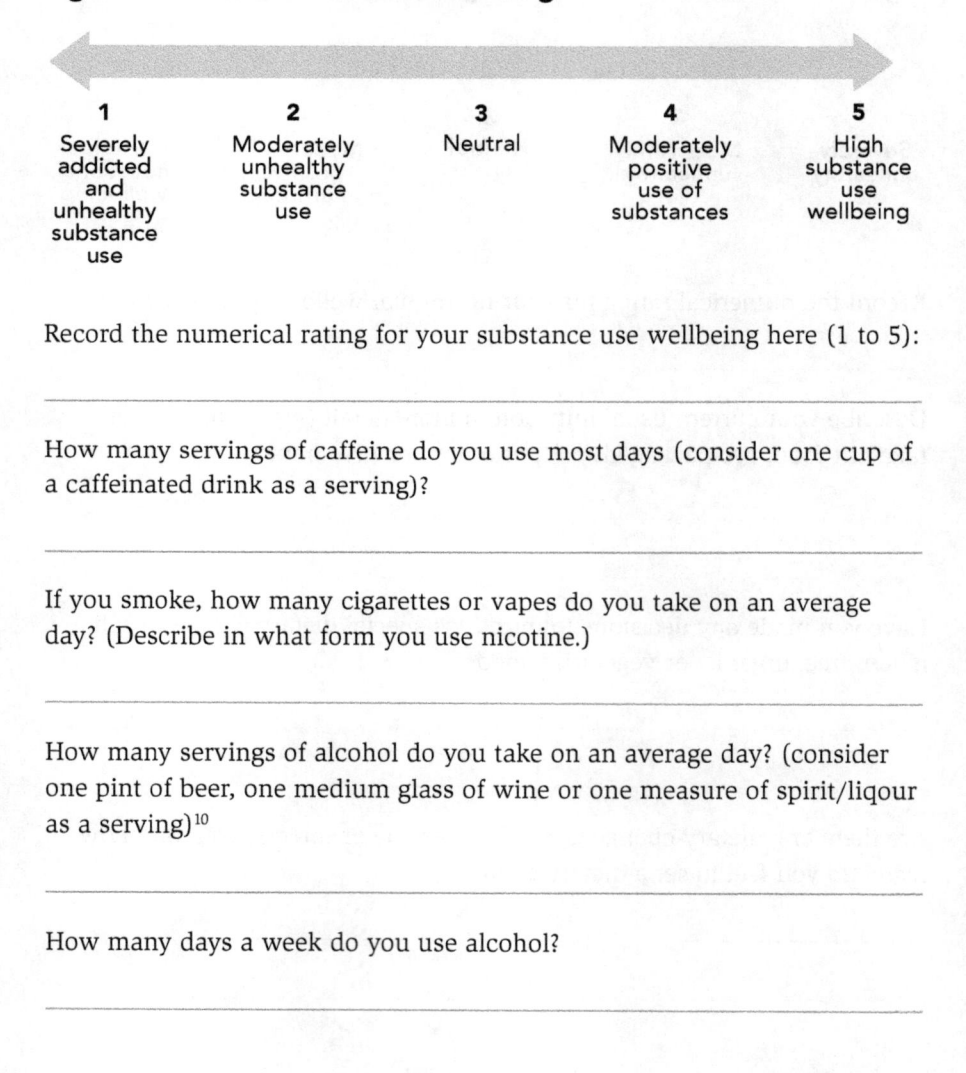

1	2	3	4	5
Severely addicted and unhealthy substance use	Moderately unhealthy substance use	Neutral	Moderately positive use of substances	High substance use wellbeing

Record the numerical rating for your substance use wellbeing here (1 to 5):

_____

How many servings of caffeine do you use most days (consider one cup of a caffeinated drink as a serving)?

_____

If you smoke, how many cigarettes or vapes do you take on an average day? (Describe in what form you use nicotine.)

_____

How many servings of alcohol do you take on an average day? (consider one pint of beer, one medium glass of wine or one measure of spirit/liqour as a serving)[10]

_____

How many days a week do you use alcohol?

_____

---

10   For a more exact definition of servings of alcohol, consider these online sources:
     National Health Service. (no date). Drink less alcohol. https://www.nhs.uk/better-health/drink-less/ (accessed March 2025)
     National Institute on Alcohol Abuse and Alcoholism. (2025). The basics: Defining how much alcohol is too much. https://www.niaaa.nih.gov/health-professionals-communities/core-resource-on-alcohol/basics-defining-how-much-alcohol-too-much (accessed March 2025)

Do you use recreational drugs, such as marijuana, cocaine, or heroin? (Describe which you use.)

How many days a week do you use recreational drugs?

Do you observe any negative effects from your substance use?

How ready do you feel to set a change goal about your use of caffeine, nicotine, alcohol, or recreational drugs?

Chapter 13: Completing your Pathways Assessment

Assessment Six: Sleep wellbeing

What is your current level of sleep wellbeing?

Figure 13.6: Sleep wellbeing

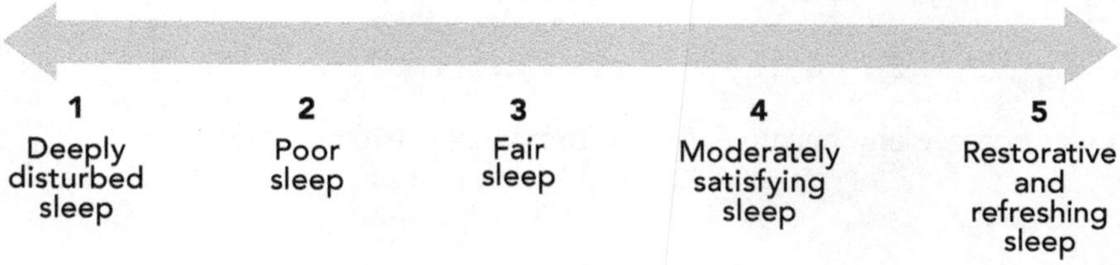

⟵─────────────────────────⟶

1	2	3	4	5
Deeply disturbed sleep	Poor sleep	Fair sleep	Moderately satisfying sleep	Restorative and refreshing sleep

Record the numerical rating for your sleep wellbeing here (1 to 5):

_____

Describe sleep difficulties (sleep onset problems, frequent awakening, early morning awakening, restless sleep, non-restorative sleep):

_____

_____

Describe any factors that disrupt your sleep or help you to sleep better:

_____

_____

Assessment Seven: Social/relationship wellbeing

What is your current level of social/relationship wellbeing?

Figure 13.7: Social/relationship wellbeing

1	2	3	4	5
Severe isolation, conflict, loneliness	Poor relationships and supports	Neutral	Moderately satisfying	Abundant social and relationship supports

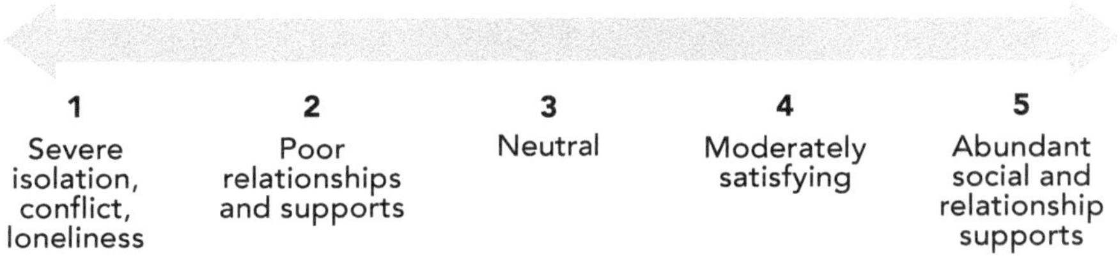

Record the numerical rating for your social/relationship wellbeing here (1 to 5):

Which relationships are your most supportive and affirming?

Are there clubs, churches, or organizations that provide you with helpful social support?

Do you have someone to call or meet with if you are upset or just need to talk?

Assessment Eight: Spiritual wellbeing

What is your current level of spiritual wellbeing?

Figure 13.8: Spiritual wellbeing

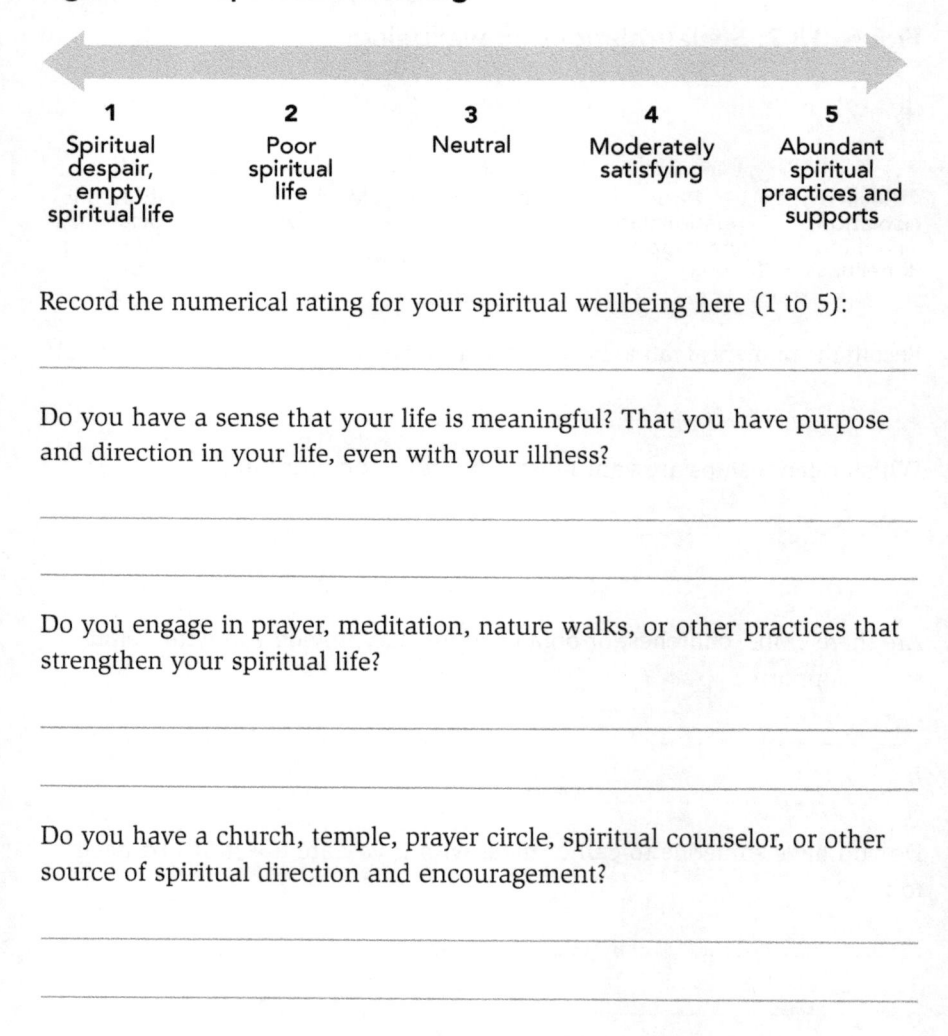

1	2	3	4	5
Spiritual despair, empty spiritual life	Poor spiritual life	Neutral	Moderately satisfying	Abundant spiritual practices and supports

Record the numerical rating for your spiritual wellbeing here (1 to 5):

Do you have a sense that your life is meaningful? That you have purpose and direction in your life, even with your illness?

Do you engage in prayer, meditation, nature walks, or other practices that strengthen your spiritual life?

Do you have a church, temple, prayer circle, spiritual counselor, or other source of spiritual direction and encouragement?

Resources

Prochaska, J. O., & Prochaska, J. M. (2016). *Changing to Thrive: Using the stages of change to overcome the top threats to your health and happiness.* Hazelden Publishing.

Assessment Nine: Illness self-management

What is your current level of illness self-management?

Quality of life for people with a long-term illness or a long-term medical condition is usually improved when they become engaged in their own healthcare, health decisions, and activities to manage the illness. Self-management might mean monitoring blood sugar and adjusting diet, taking exercise or yoga classes to improve physical fitness, or making dietary changes for better health.

Figure 13.9: Illness self-management

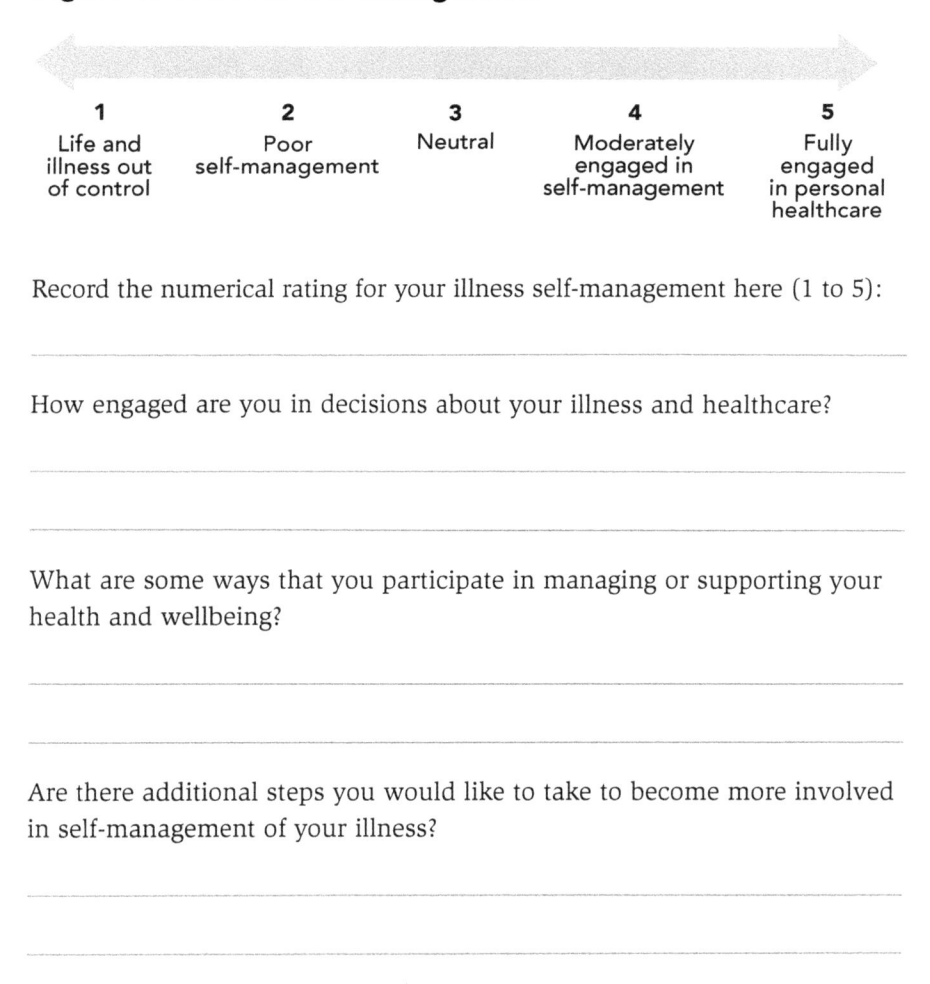

1	2	3	4	5
Life and illness out of control	Poor self-management	Neutral	Moderately engaged in self-management	Fully engaged in personal healthcare

Record the numerical rating for your illness self-management here (1 to 5):

How engaged are you in decisions about your illness and healthcare?

What are some ways that you participate in managing or supporting your health and wellbeing?

Are there additional steps you would like to take to become more involved in self-management of your illness?

Assessment Ten: Readiness for change

What is your current level of readiness for change?

This is probably the most important part of the Pathways Model. What is your general readiness for change? Are you reading this book because someone else is pressuring you to make changes, or are you personally ready to make changes? James Prochaska developed the stages of change model, which rates individuals according to their current readiness for change. According to his model, there are five stages of change:

- **Pre-contemplation** – not currently motivated to make changes, not even thinking about it.
- **Contemplation** – open to information, thinking about changes, but not ready to start.
- **Preparation/determination** – ready to plan changes and mentally determined to act.
- **Action** – taking steps, making changes.
- **Maintenance** – monitoring one's condition, and ready to make further steps to maintain changes.

If you are stuck at the pre-contemplation stage, it is better not to set a specific goal. You might fail to act on the goal and then judge yourself as a failure. It is better to see your actual readiness and focus your energy on improving your readiness as the first step.

Figure 13.10: Readiness for change

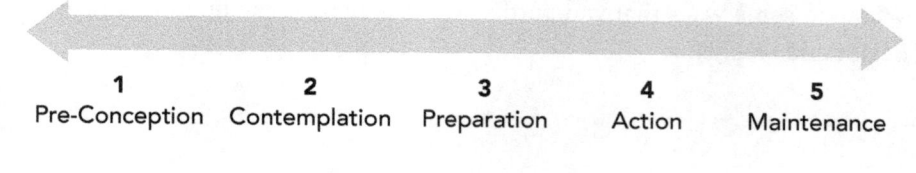

1	2	3	4	5
Pre-Conception	Contemplation	Preparation	Action	Maintenance

Record the numerical rating for your readiness for change here (1 to 5):

_____

In the following lines, describe your subjective feelings of readiness for change overall:

_____

Is there any knowledge, any information, or any preliminary preparation you could make, that might help you to feel readier for action?

Is there anyone who could assist you to tackle some change goals, and are you ready to ask this person for help? Do not be ashamed of asking for help. Part of practical wisdom is creating the best conditions for us to succeed in our goals. Often sharing lifestyle goals with a friend or family member can help individuals reach success:

Sometimes, people feel more ready to make changes in one area than another. Describe any areas where you feel more ready to act:

Chapter 13: Completing your Pathways Assessment

Conclusion: Your Pathways Assessment Graph

You have created a numerical rating in each of the ten assessment areas. Now take those ten ratings and insert them in the following graph, which will create a picture of your overall wellbeing. You can use this graph to guide you as you design your Pathways program. It makes sense to choose some goals that will strengthen areas where your wellbeing ratings are lower.

Each bar in this graph represents a rating for one Pathways Assessment area, on a scale from one to five (with one indicating very low and five indicating very high wellbeing). Color in your own rating for each area.

Figure 13.11: Pathways Assessment Graph in ten lifestyle areas

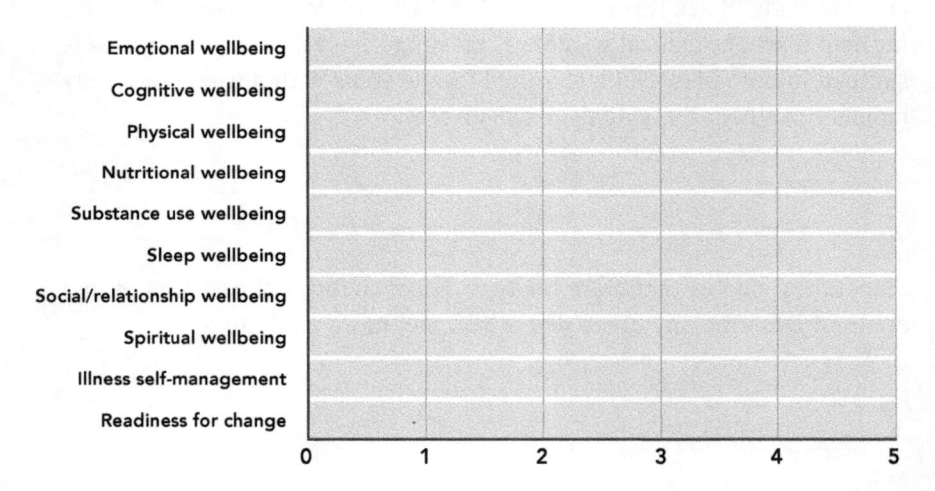

Area	Rating (0–5)
Emotional wellbeing	
Cognitive wellbeing	
Physical wellbeing	
Nutritional wellbeing	
Substance use wellbeing	
Sleep wellbeing	
Social/relationship wellbeing	
Spiritual wellbeing	
Illness self-management	
Readiness for change	

Final message: *The Pathways Assessment provides an assessment of your wellbeing across ten areas. It examines your health risks and wellbeing across these areas, ending with a realistic evaluation of your readiness for change. This overall picture of your health risks and strengths will guide you as you set Level One, Two, and Three goals.*

Chapter 14:
Selecting Level One goals

Summary: Level One in the Pathways Model involves setting self-directed goals for new self-care practices, reducing health-risk behaviors, and increasing health-enhancing lifestyle elements. Chronic stress, long-term illness, and the accompanying emotions disturb biological rhythms; the Level One steps restore these rhythms. Once goals are set, individuals are encouraged to review their progress regularly and reset goals as needed for optimal success.

Keywords: Pathways Model, goal setting, Level One, self-care, lifestyle, health-risk behaviors, biological rhythms

Approaching Level One

In Level One, you are invited to set small initial goals, involving self-directed wellness activities. Possible Level One steps include increasing movement, practicing paced diaphragmatic breathing, correcting poor nutrition, reducing stress levels, self-quieting activities, and restoring healthier sleep patterns. Here are some Level One options for you:

- Paced diaphragmatic breathing
- Dietary changes
- Improving sleep habits/sleep hygiene

- Walking short distances
- Reduce everyday exposure to stress
- Moving with music
- Praying
- Sitting quietly
- Playing guitar or piano

Consider now which Level One goals you might like to adopt at this time. Usually, it is practical to choose two or three. You are also free to consider other possible self-guided initial goals, as long as they are simple and will move you toward overall wellness. You can always add additional Level One goals later or change a goal if you find you are not progressing well with it.

Level One goal setting

Level One, goal 1: _____

Goal 1 – Time of day and duration:

_____

Goal 1 – Times per week:

_____

Level One, goal 2: _____

Goal 2 – Time of day and duration:

_____

Goal 2 – Times per week:

_____

Level One, goal 3: _____

Goal 3 – Time of day and duration:

_____

Goal 3 – Times per week:

_____

Level One weekly progress on goals

Each week, it is valuable to review your progress on your Level One goals, consider any obstacles, and reset goals if necessary. It can be helpful to do this on Sunday afternoon or evening, reviewing progress over the past week, and re-committing for the new week.

Progress on Level One, goal 1

This week, I accomplished the following on goal 1:

Possible obstacles to this goal include:

Next week, I plan to adjust the goal as follows:

Progress on Level One, goal 2

This week, I accomplished the following on goal 2:

Possible obstacles to this goal include:

Next week, I plan to adjust the goal as follows:

Progress on Level One, goal 3

This week, I accomplished the following on goal 3:

_____

_____

Possible obstacles to this goal include:

_____

_____

Next week, I plan to adjust the goal as follows:

_____

_____

I have decided to add the following goal for the coming week:

Level One, goal 4: _____

Goal 4 – Time of day and duration:

_____

Goal 4 – Times per week:

_____

Four-week review

Every four weeks it is useful to conduct a larger review, assessing the impact of your Level One activities on your overall wellbeing.

Self-rating of your engagement on these goals

In the following lines, assess how much you have felt involved with these Level One goals and lifestyle changes:

What is the impact of these wellness activities on you as a person, on your physical symptoms, on your emotions, and on your self-experience?

Given your experience so far, do you believe you would benefit most from continuing these goals in exactly the same way for the next month, changing them, or even starting Level One over again with new goals?

How ready do you feel to move to Level Two and add higher-level goals? Be honest with yourself, as it is often better to stay longer with Level One until you feel entirely ready to move to the next level:

Final message: *Level One guides the individual to set self-directed goals for self-care and lifestyle change. These goals serve to restore biological rhythms, to moderate distress and suffering related to your illness or health conditions, and at times to reduce the intensity and frequency of symptoms. Level One also builds the individual's confidence that self-directed changes can impact health, wellbeing, and quality of life. It is worthwhile continuing with some Level One self-care practices as you move ahead to Level Two.*

Chapter 15:
Selecting Level Two goals

Summary: Level Two in the Pathways Model involves acquiring new self-regulation skills, coping skills, and self-care practices. This level frequently involves using available resources such as written instructions, educational CDs, apps, podcasts, and community-based classes. Level Two interventions such as emotional journaling and mindfulness practices also contribute to emotional healing.

Keywords: : Pathways Model, Level Two, goal setting, coping skills, community resources, educational materials

Approaching Level Two

In Level Two, you are invited to choose higher-level goals, such as acquiring self-care skills, coping skills, and health-enhancing practices. In Level Two, you may benefit from written instructions, relevant books and articles, educational CDs, podcasts, and apps. Level Two self-care or coping skills include progressive muscle relaxation, autogenic training, meditation, and guided imagery. You may also benefit from community resources such as yoga centres, mindfulness classes, meditation groups, and similar supports offering health-enhancing activities in groups or solo training. Here is a list of possible Level Two options for you:

Chapter 15: Selecting Level Two goals

- Progressive muscle relaxation
- Autogenic training
- Heart rate variability
- The pause
- Assertiveness: setting limits
- Mindfulness training
- Emotional journaling
- Guided imagery
- 12-step groups
- Meditation practices
- Prayer groups
- Yoga
- Qigong
- Tai-Chi
- Aquatherapy

The appendices to this book provide many resources to help you understand and implement Level Two. Appendix A includes instructions for several Level Two self-care and coping skills. Appendix B includes helpful YouTube videos, books, CDs, and DVDs to guide self-care and lifestyle change. Appendix C provides Worksheets for Healing Pathways. Illness is always accompanied by emotional challenges and, in turn, emotional struggles aggravate illness. The Appendix C worksheets are designed to improve your self-awareness of your emotional struggles, and to suggest resources for managing these struggles.

> *"In Level Two, you are invited to choose higher level goals, such as acquiring self-care skills, coping skills, and health enhancing practices."*

Level Two goal setting

Consider which Level Two goals you wish to adopt at this time. Usually, it is practical to choose two or three goals. You are encouraged to consider lifestyle choices, skills, and practices you have read about or even learned, but not applied regularly in your life.

Feel free to continue some or all of your Level One goals, if they still seem beneficial. However, if any of these goals absorb too much of your available time and energy, you will need to eliminate that goal, or reduce how many times a week you practice it, in order to have time and energy for Level Two.

Level Two, goal 1: _____

Goal 1 – Guidance, resources, instructions, other sources:

Goal 1 – Schedule and frequency:

Level Two, goal 2: _____

Goal 2 – Guidance, resources, instructions, other sources:

Goal 2 – Schedule and frequency:

Level Two, goal 3: _____

Goal 3 – Guidance, resources, instructions, other sources:

Goal 3 – Schedule and frequency:

Level Two weekly progress on goals

Each week, it is valuable to review your progress on your Level Two goals, consider any obstacles, and reset goals if necessary. It can be helpful to do this on Sunday afternoon or evening, reviewing progress over the past week, and re-committing for the new week.

Progress on Level Two, goal 1

This week, I accomplished the following on goal 1:

_____

_____

Possible obstacles to this goal include:

_____

_____

Next week, I plan to adjust the goal as follows:

_____

_____

Progress on Level Two, goal 2

This week, I accomplished the following on goal 2:

_____

_____

Possible obstacles to this goal include:

_____

_____

Next week, I plan to adjust the goal as follows:

_____

_____

Progress on Level Two, goal 3

This week, I accomplished the following on goal 3:

_____

_____

Possible obstacles to this goal include:

_____

_____

Next week, I plan to adjust the goal as follows:

_____

_____

I have decided to add the following goal for the coming week:

Level Two, goal 4: _____

Goal 4 – Guidance, resources, instructions, other sources:

_____

Goal 4 – Schedule and frequency:

_____

> *"Each week, it is valuable to review progress on Level Two goals, consider any obstacles, and reset goals if necessary."*

Four-week review

Every four weeks it is useful to conduct a larger review, assessing the impact of your Level Two activities on your overall wellbeing.

Self-rating of your engagement on Level Two goals

In the following lines, assess how much you have felt involved with these Level Two goals and lifestyle changes:

_____

_____

What is the impact of these wellness activities on you as a person, on your physical symptoms, on your emotions, and on your self-experience?

_____

_____

Given your experience so far, do you believe you would benefit most from continuing these goals in exactly the same way for the next month, changing them, or even starting Level Two over again with new goals?

_____

_____

How ready do you feel to move to Level Three and add higher-level goals? Be honest, as it is often better to stay longer with Level One and Level Two activities until you feel entirely ready to move to the next level:

_____

_____

Healing themes at Level Two

What is the emotional experience for you of living with long-term illness? There are many common emotional experiences reported by individuals:

- Anger
- Anxiety
- Fear of the unknown
- Frustration
- Self-blame
- Loss of control

- Sadness
- Sense of loss
- Shame and embarrassment
- Despondency and despair
- Spiritual doubts

Many individuals pursuing the Pathways Model report experiences of emotional healing and rebirth of hope. Simply carrying out self-care practices and wellness-oriented lifestyle changes often brings a sense of self-efficacy. Self-efficacy is the experience that you can do something positive for yourself and it will make a difference.

Many of the Level Two activities also directly aid emotional healing. For example, emotional journaling can be painful, yet journaling over several days or weeks often leads to a reduction in the intensity of painful emotions and an upsurge in positive emotions. Mindfulness practices can also transform emotions within weeks. Appendix C provides Healing Pathways Worksheets, designed to enhance awareness of emotional struggles that accompany long-term illness, and to highlight pathways to manage these struggles.

> *"Simply carrying out self-care practices and wellness-oriented lifestyle changes often brings a sense of self-efficacy. Self-efficacy is the experience that you can do something positive for yourself and it will make a difference."*

In a previous book, Dr. Moss described the story of a woman with multiple sclerosis (MS), who had to make major life changes due to MS-related disabilities.[11] She experienced a deep despair about the loss of her previous life. Yet mindfulness practices transformed this despair, allowing her to observe and accept it. She concluded that it was reasonable and healthy to feel distress over her losses, and realized she could live with her now accepted feelings.

> **Final message:** *Level Two guides individuals to acquire new self-regulation skills and engage in health-enhancing lifestyle changes. Level Two activities also draw on electronic resources and community-based groups and classes. Many people will continue with some Level One and Level Two activities, as long as they still have time and energy to fully engage in their new Level Three treatments.*

---

11 Khazan, I., & Moss, D. (Eds.) (2020). *Mindfulness, Acceptance, and Compassion in Biofeedback Practice*. Association for Applied Psychophysiology and Biofeedback.

Chapter 16:

Selecting Level Three treatments and professionals

> **Summary:** Level Three in the Pathways Model includes professional interventions, ranging from psychotherapy to physical therapy, and from acupuncture to medical management. Level Three treatments address remaining areas of health-risk behaviors, and provide targeted interventions to manage symptoms of long-term illness. Level Three treatments can also be selected specifically for their impact on continuing emotional distress. This chapter aids the individual in selecting therapies and the healthcare professionals who will provide them.
>
> **Keywords:** Pathways Model, Level Three, choosing interventions, choosing a practitioner

Approaching Level Three

Level Three in the Pathways Model includes professional interventions – services provided by a health practitioner, such as biofeedback, hypnosis, energy therapy, psychotherapy, physical therapy, acupuncture, or medication management. Most Pathways Model clients use at least two or three Level Three therapies in the same period. We recommend more than one professional intervention simultaneously for two reasons. First, there is not yet enough reliable research evidence to tell us which of the available treatments will provide the greatest benefit for any single person. Second, in integrative healthcare, we find benefit in *synergy*: two or more interventions often augment each other's positive effects.

Choosing the best Level Three interventions for your Pathways program

Think for a moment about your long-term conditions and/or long-term illnesses. Are you more impacted in movement, emotion, or thinking? Think about your Pathways Assessment Graph. Do you have less overall wellbeing in movement areas, nutrition, social supports, or spiritual resources? Are you suffering more with pain, sick feelings, anxiety, or discouragement? Are you more concerned about being ill, losing your quality of life, or not being able to do activities you enjoy? It makes sense to consider a Level Three therapy that is often helpful in areas where your wellbeing is lower and areas where you have symptoms.

Level Three therapies

- Hypnosis
- Biofeedback and neurofeedback
- Psychotherapy
- Physical therapy
- Energy therapies (Reiki)
- Body work/somatic therapies
- Therapeutic massage
- Acupuncture
- Meditation trainers
- Spiritual counseling
- Psychiatric care
- Medical management

The following professional treatments can often be helpful with **pain, headache, and restricted movement**:

- Physical therapy
- Biofeedback
- Hypnosis
- Acupuncture
- Therapeutic massage
- Somatic therapies
- Medical management by a pain specialist

The following professional treatments and self-care practices are often helpful with **anxiety, depression, and emotional disorders**:

- Psychotherapy and counseling
- Hypnosis
- Biofeedback
- Emotional journaling
- Mindfulness-oriented therapies
- Energy medicine
- Psychiatry

The following professional treatments and self-care practices are often helpful with **general distress related to life with long-term illness**, which may not qualify as an emotional disorder:

- Acceptance and Commitment Therapy (ACT)
- Compassion Focused Therapy (CFT)
- Heart rate variability training
- Hypnosis
- Mindfulness-oriented therapies
- Meditation training
- Emotional journaling

The following professional treatments are often helpful with **disturbed sleep**:

- Cognitive behavioral therapy for insomnia (CBT-I)
- Hypnosis
- Guided imagery
- Nutrition

The following professional treatments are helpful with **spiritual conflicts and troubles**:

- Spiritually based psychotherapy
- Meditation training
- Pastoral counseling

Chapter 16: Selecting Level Three treatments and professionals

The following professional treatments are often helpful with **nausea, sick feelings, recurrent fever, and inflammation**:

- Nutritional counseling
- Hypnosis
- Acupuncture
- Energy medicine
- Medical management

For habit change – including smoking cessation, dietary change, or increasing exercise – we recommend a life coach with experience in habit change, along with a recognised healthcare practitioner such as a substance abuse counselor, dietician, or physical therapist. Sometimes, a hypnotherapist or psychologist can also improve your success in habit change, by helping you better manage emotions that drive your addictive or destructive behaviors.

Choosing a specific practitioner

It is not always easy to choose the best possible practitioners, especially in lesser-known areas such as nutrition and energy medicine. The first choice is to use a healthcare professional who is trained and certified in a speciality area relevant to your condition. For example, for Americans, we would rather refer our clients to a hypnosis practitioner who is first a licensed health practitioner, and second certified by the most respected professional organizations, the American Society of Clinical Hypnosis and the Society for Clinical and Experimental Hypnosis. For UK residents, we would recommend accredited practitioners who are trained by a body such as the British Society of Clinical Hypnosis. Or, to take another example, we would rather refer patients for dietary guidance to a certified nutrition specialist or a registered dietician who is also trained by the Institute for Functional Medicine (IFM).

Sometimes, however, a strong recommendation from a trusted source can be more important than the specific licence or certification. If your doctor knows that a nutritionist has been helpful to many people with long-term illness, for example, that can make up for the lack of IFM training.

Most important is that you want a Level Three professional who treats you with respect, takes time to talk at each session, and shares knowledge about your illness and available treatment options. In addition, your Level Three therapists should communicate regularly with your primary care physician, and with any professional who is coordinating your Pathways program. If you are managing your own Pathways program, that means the Level Three therapist must report any new findings and observations directly to you.

Further, your Level Three professionals work for you. You have a right to change practitioners, request a change in the treatment, and even stop the treatment if you are not satisfied. However, we encourage you to not give up too soon. Remember that many complementary or mind-body treatments involve learning skills or adjusting a delicate long-term balance in your body. Allow adequate time to see the long-term benefits. Nevertheless, you have the right to decide to stop treatments or change practitioners.

> *"You have a right to change practitioners, request a change in the treatment, and even stop the treatment if you are not satisfied."*

Level Three treatment selection

Level Three treatment 1

Practitioner name: _____

    Treatment 1 – Description:

    _____

    Treatment 1 – Resources, instructions, sources of guidance:

    _____

    Treatment 1 – Times per week:

    _____

Level Three treatment 2

Practitioner name: _____

    Treatment 2 – Description:

    _____

    Treatment 2 – Resources, instructions, sources of guidance:

    _____

    Treatment 2 – Times per week:

    _____

Level Three treatment 3

Practitioner name: _____

    Treatment 3 – Description:

    _____

    Treatment 3 – Resources, instructions, sources of guidance:

    _____

    Treatment 3 – Times per week:

    _____

Level Three weekly progress in treatment

Each week, it is valuable to review your progress on your Level Three goals, consider any obstacles, and reset goals if necessary. It can be helpful to do this on Sunday afternoon or evening, reviewing progress over the past week, and re-committing for the new week.

Progress on Level Three treatment 1

This week, I accomplished the following on treatment 1:

Possible obstacles to this treatment include:

Next week, I plan to adjust my use of the treatment as follows:

Progress on Level Three treatment 2

This week, I accomplished the following on treatment 2:

Possible obstacles to this treatment include:

Next week, I plan to adjust my use of the treatment as follows:

Progress on Level Three treatment 3

This week, I accomplished the following on treatment 3:

_____

_____

Possible obstacles to this treatment include:

_____

_____

Next week, I plan to adjust my use of the treatment as follows:

_____

_____

I have decided to add the following treatment for the coming month:

Level Three treatment 4

Practitioner name: _____

Treatment 4 – Description:

_____

Treatment 4 – Resources, instructions, sources of guidance:

_____

Treatment 4 – Times per week:

_____

Four-week review

Every four weeks it is useful to conduct a larger review, assessing the impact of your Level Three treatments and activities on your overall wellbeing.

Self-rating of your engagement on Level Three treatments

In the following lines, assess how much you have felt involved with the Level Three treatments and any related lifestyle changes:

What is the impact of these treatments on you as a person, on your physical symptoms, on your emotions, and on your self-experience?

Given your experience so far, do you believe you would benefit most from continuing these goals in exactly the same way for the next month, changing them, or even starting Level Three over again with new goals?

How ready do you feel to end the formal treatment in Level Three for now and shift to long-term self-care and well lifestyle? Be honest, as it is often better to stay longer with Level Three treatments until you feel entirely ready to move to a more self-directed lifestyle. Of course, you can always return to any Level Three treatment again in the future and try new treatments as well. Managing long-term health conditions is a lifelong process.

Afterword: maintenance

The Pathways Model can only ever be as successful as the individual who is implementing it. It is easy to become discouraged with long-term health conditions, or with setbacks in self-care. Please remember that setbacks are normal. The success of the Pathways Model depends on you assessing what went wrong, rebounding, maintaining the growth mindset, and revising your goals.

Progress when using integrative and complementary therapies often follows a "sawtooth curve", resembling the blade of a saw. This means that your condition will probably be up and down each day or week, with progress followed by setbacks. Yet if the therapies you have selected are beneficial for you, that sawtooth curve will gradually trend upward, despite the day-to-day fluctuations (See Figure 1.)

Figure 16.1: Sawtooth curve

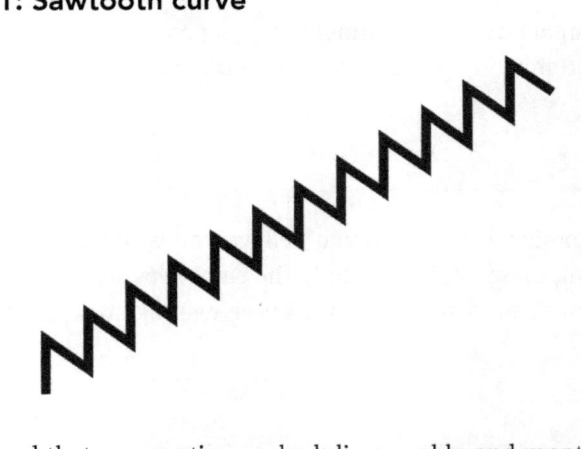

We recommend that you continue scheduling weekly and monthly Pathways reviews, and continually assess which Pathways self-care and lifestyle elements you use most regularly, and which seem to provide the most benefit.

It is also helpful to repeat the entire Pathways Assessment process introduced in Chapter 13 at least every six months, producing a new Pathways Assessment Graph. The nature of long-term illness is that you may be challenged by your health condition for a prolonged period of time or even lifelong, so periodic reassessments are valuable to evaluate your progress and guide you in shifting goals over time. The Pathways Assessment Graph can guide you to reset new Level One and Two goals or even to initiate a new Level Three treatment.

At this moment, which self-care and lifestyle elements seem most important and relevant to demand your time and energy?

At this moment, which community resources, classes and groups seem most beneficial and comfortable for you to continue now and indefinitely?

At this moment, are there any additional self-care practices or supports that you believe you need for yourself, to maintain your full engagement in a lifelong Pathways self-management program?

Looking forward, are there Level Three treatments that you already know you want to return to quickly if you lose progress and suffer setbacks?

Final message: *Level Three includes treatments provided by healthcare professionals, ranging from psychotherapy to acupuncture. Long-term health conditions create long-term challenges, often with intermittent periods of more severe symptoms. Individuals in the Pathways Model will usually continue elements of Level One and Level Two activity long term, and periodically resume Level Three treatments.*

Appendix A:
Instructions for self-care skills

This appendix includes Pathways Skill Modules with written instructions to guide you in learning a variety of self-care skills, including mindful breathing, autogenic training, visualizing a calm scene, expressive writing, a mantra meditation, mindfulness training, informal mindfulness meditation, a special mindfulness exercise, progressive muscle relaxation, and self-hypnosis. In each case, read through the instructions several times, until you achieve a good understanding of the exercise. Then use the written instructions to guide you through it. Each exercise begins on a new page, to make it easier to reproduce the instructions for your use.

Each of these exercises involves a form of self-regulation. You are engaged in regulating your own mind and emotions. You remain in control and direct your own experience. If a specific exercise is comfortable for you, continue with it. If any exercise, or some aspect of it, is uncomfortable or causes distress, use your own imagination to modify the experience for yourself. You are free to stop the exercise at any time.

Some of these Skill Modules were adapted with changes from a previous publication by Donald Moss and Fredric Shaffer, *A Primer of Biofeedback*, with kind permission of the publisher, the Association for Applied Psychophysiology and Biofeedback.[12]

---

[12] Adapted with permission from D. Moss, & F. Shaffer (2022). Chapter 9. Adjunctive interventions for biofeedback practice. *A Primer of biofeedback*. (pp. 83-97). Association for Applied Psychophysiology and Biofeedback.

Chapter 16: Selecting Level Three treatments and professionals

Skill Module 1: Mindful breathing

Mindful breathing is an important tool for creating a relaxed state of body, mind, and spirit. The first objective of mindful breathing is to create a relaxed process of breathing, which is smooth, gentle, and effortless. The second objective is to absorb one's mind fully in the process of breathing, leaving behind the stress of life, the pressure of schedules, and the burdens of life.

Mindful breathing is focused on the diaphragm, the abdomen, and not the chest. The diaphragm is a dome-shaped muscle between the lungs and the abdominal cavity. Each time you inhale, the diaphragm contracts and flattens its curve, creating a vacuum into which the lungs can expand. As this happens the diaphragm pushes the abdominal muscles outward. Watch the stomach of a baby rise and fall as it breathes and you will see this natural process in action. Many adults, because of tension, illness, or the desire to have a thin, flat waist, will resist this natural movement. Breathing exercises can assist us to re-learn the gentle natural breathing of the infant.

Instructions

Mindful breathing can be practiced in any position. It is easiest to begin when you are most relaxed, lying on the floor. Lie on your back with your arms at your sides. Turn your palms upwards. Many people find it easier to relax the diaphragm if they bend their knees, placing their feet flat on the floor.

Relax your body completely, especially the stomach and abdomen. Now, breathe comfortably, fully, and slowly, concentrating on the diaphragm, and feeling your stomach rise as you inhale and fall as you exhale. Relax the abdominal muscles more and more completely, using the diaphragm, and not the stomach muscles, to create the rise and fall of the abdomen.

Each time you inhale, slowly and gently take in a full breath. Enlarge the volume of air in the inhalation, yet do not force the breath in an uncomfortable way. Pause for a moment, then begin to exhale.

Exhale fully, emptying out slowly and smoothly. Allow the exhalation phase to stretch out longer than the inhalation. The exhalation phase is the moment of maximal release of tensions, and in relaxation should usually be longer than the inhalation. For most people, a ratio of exhale-time to inhale-time of about two to one is optimal. But if that is uncomfortable, accept your own preference. The two-to-one ratio is not essential.

With each inhalation, the sympathetic nervous system activates, and our heart rate increases; with each exhalation, the parasympathetic nervous system becomes dominant, and heart rate slows.

After each exhalation, pause briefly again, and then resume inhaling.

Generally, it is optimal to breathe in through the nostrils and out through the mouth. However, if you are congested or otherwise uncomfortable breathing in through the nostrils, then inhale through the mouth. As you exhale, purse your lips to create a slight resistance to the flow of air. Form a circle with your lips and feel the flow of breath as you exhale.

You will notice that as you breathe in a mindful and relaxed fashion, each breath will become larger, involving a larger volume of air, and your rate of breathing will decrease. For effective relaxation, a breathing rate of about six breaths a minute is optimal, but it is equally important that your breathing remains smooth, gentle, and without effort. Any straining and effort to breathe correctly will diminish the positive effects of breath training.

You are exercising the muscle of the diaphragm each time you practice this exercise. As it becomes stronger and more mobile, the diaphragm will spontaneously participate more fully in your normal breathing.

With each inhale, notice a slight increase in abdominal muscle tension. With each exhale, you will experience a release of tensions.

Take each breath gently and without effort. Enjoy breathing in a relaxed fashion. Bring your attention to the process of breathing. Gently notice distractions, accept them, and bring your mind back to breathing.

After several minutes of practice on the floor, you can sit in any comfortable position and continue mindful breathing. You may find this a little harder at first, but you'll soon catch on. It helps to close your eyes and concentrate on relaxing the stomach, allowing it to swell outward and relax back inward. Once you know how to breathe correctly, you can practice mindful breathing wherever you are. It may take a couple of weeks to train yourself, but you will find the results well worth the effort.

Remember the element of mindfulness. The principle of mindfulness is to pay attention in a very special way, absorbing yourself fully, without judging or criticizing. Regardless of how you are breathing at this moment, enjoy absorbing your attention fully in the process of breathing.

Experiment with placing a weight, such as a large book, a bag of rice, or even your own hand, over your abdomen to increase your awareness of the breathing process and the movement of your abdomen.

When distracting thoughts arise, notice them, accept them mindfully, and return your attention to the process of breathing. Be aware of the entire cycle of breathing, following the initial inhalation into your body, through the airways and into the lungs. Experience the slow movement of your diaphragm as you inhale. Then continue absorbing yourself fully with the breathing process as you empty out the lungs and exhale this volume of air through your mouth.

Breathing fully and deeply forms the foundation for many relaxation skills and spiritual exercises. Many ancient traditions identify breath with life and with the human spirit. In Genesis 2:7, God breathed a breath of life into Adam's nostrils, and "thus man became a living being". The Latin word *inspirare* (to breathe) has the same root as *spiritus* (spirit), and the Greek word *pneuma* refers to a breath and also to the soul or spirit.

Practical guidelines

Remind yourself to breathe mindfully, diaphragmatically, gently, and fully as you begin any relaxation or meditation exercise.

There are many available aids to guide your breathing practice. Breath training apps available for the smart phone or tablet include Breathe2Relax, Breathing Zone, and the Inner Balance.

Skill Module 2: Autogenic training

Autogenic training (AT) is a self-regulation technique that produces profound relaxation and relief from the negative effects of stress. "Autogenic" means "generated from within". The German Johann Schultz developed this procedure in the 1920s and 1930s, and his colleague Wolfgang Luthe brought it to the attention of the English-speaking world.

AT mobilizes our innate ability for healing and recuperation. AT consists of a series of simple, easily learned mental exercises that link mind and body together in association with deep relaxation. These exercises allow the mind and body to become calm by switching off the body's stress responses.

Once learned, AT is a useful life skill, providing the inner resources to maintain a healthy balance and deal with stress in body and mind. AT has been successfully used clinically to alleviate insomnia, panic attacks, high blood pressure, asthma, phobias, irritable bowel, migraine, and many other conditions. Many people also learn the method to improve efficiency, mobilize creativity, and achieve a higher state of wellbeing.

Instructions

Adopt a passive mental attitude – an attitude of letting go or letting be. Remind yourself to set aside all problems and effort during this time of relaxation, and to maintain a detached but alert state of mind. If you are distracted by intrusive thoughts or worries, let the distractions be there. You don't need to fight with these thoughts. Being distracted is normal during learning. Gently bring yourself back to the relaxation practice.

Mentally repeat each autogenic phrase to yourself, beginning with phrase A. Don't try to *make* anything happen; rather, allow yourself to imagine what the sensation might be like. Effort blocks relaxation. Passively allowing the sensations is more effective.

Exercise 1: "I experience heaviness in my limbs."
A. My right arm is heavy, comfortably and pleasantly heavy.
B. My left arm is heavy, comfortably and pleasantly heavy.
C. My right leg is heavy, comfortably and pleasantly heavy.
D. My left leg is heavy, comfortably and pleasantly heavy.
E. My entire body is becoming heavier and heavier, comfortably and pleasantly heavy.

Exercise 2: "I experience my limbs becoming loose, limp, and comfortably relaxed."

A. My right arm is loose and limp.

B. My left arm is loose and limp.

C. My right leg is loose, limp, and comfortably relaxed.

D. My left leg is loose, limp, and comfortably relaxed.

Exercise 3: "I experience warmth in my limbs."

A. My right arm is warm, comfortably warm.

B. My left arm is warm, comfortably warm.

C. My right leg is warm, comfortably warm.

D. My left leg is warm, comfortably warm.

Exercise 4: "My heartbeat is calm and relaxed."

A. With each breath I take, my heartbeat becomes calmer and slower and relaxed.

B. My heartbeat is calm and relaxed, slow, calm, and relaxed.

Note: The original scripts provided by Schultz and Luthe suggested that the heart becomes "regular". However, since so many individuals today have been taught that a healthy heart is more variable, the language has been modified here to avoid confusion.

Exercise 5: "My breath flows through me. Slowly and deeply, I am breathed."[13]

A. I allow my breathing to occur automatically, without effort.

B. I allow my breathing to slow and relax.

C. I experience each phase of my breathing and its effects on my entire body-mind.

D. My breathing is smooth, gentle, and comfortably relaxed.

Exercise 6: "My solar plexus is warm."

A. I experience warmth in the solar plexus, the area just in front of the spine, below the sternum.

B. My solar plexus radiates warmth.

---

13   This phrase feels awkward in English but conveys the meaning of being passive to what happens.

Exercise 7: "My forehead is cool."

A. With each breath I take, my forehead feels cooler and more comfortable.

B. My forehead is more and more cool and more and more comfortable.

The phrases in all six standard exercises can be interspersed with the phrase: "My mind is at peace. My body is relaxed and my mind is at peace".

Practical guidelines

During autogenic training, some individuals report relaxation induced anxiety. They feel calmer, yet the light almost floaty feeling feels unfamiliar, and this may trigger anxiety. Others experience a variety of intense emotions – memories, the pain or discomfort of past illnesses, tears, and other phenomena. Accept these emotional discharges as normal and temporary parts of the relaxation and healing process. Often, the emotions are an important part of self-awareness and healing.

Sometimes during the practice of AT, your heart rate may increase. If this happens, open your eyes, sit back in your chair, and slow your breathing. In the very rare circumstance that your heart rate does not stabilize within ten minutes, consult your healthcare provider.

If you already know that you suffer tachycardia or atrial fibrillation, show this exercise to your healthcare provider and ask for advice on whether to use it. Note that some people will experience a slowing of the heart rate and a reduction in arrythmias with many kinds of relaxation exercises.

Resources

Luthe, W., & de Rivera, L. (2015). *Introductory workshop: Introduction to the methods of autogenic training, therapy, and psychotherapy.* Create Space Independent Publishing Platform.

UW Integrative Health. (no date). *Autogenic training.* School of Medicine and Public Health. University of Wisconsin, Madison. https://www.fammed.wisc.edu/files/webfm-uploads/documents/outreach/im/tool-autogenic-training.pdf (accessed February 2025).

VeryWellMind (2025). *Autogenic training for reducing anxiety.* https://www.verywellmind.com/how-to-practice-autogenic-training-for-relaxation-3024387 (accessed February 2025).

Skill Module 3: Visualizing a calm scene

Visualization and imagery claim deep roots in the spiritual traditions of humankind. Native American tribes developed complex rituals, sometimes aided by ingestion of psychedelic plants or the use of sweat lodges to facilitate visions, and vision quests that ritualize the seeking of a sense of identity, often in conjunction with identifying a totem animal. Similarly, the ancient Egyptians and Greeks used sleep temples, rituals, and visions to commune with supernatural dimensions of life, often for healing purposes.

Modern interest in imagery as a tool for mental health and medicine emerged in the 1970s and 1980s with an explosion of research on the use of mental imagery for relaxation, stress reduction, and health. Applications range from dermatology to diabetes to fibromyalgia to anxiety.

The following instructions introduce widely used visualization/imagery techniques for relaxation and stress reduction. The imagery that is most soothing varies from person to person, depending on life experience and past traumatic experiences. The beach imagery that is soothing for one patient may evoke anxiety in the next.

Instructions

Begin by selecting a place – a calm scene – that you will visit in the exercise. This can be a real place where you have spent time in the past, or entirely imaginary. It should seem soothing, safe, comfortable, and peaceful. Common places include a beach, a meadow, a log cabin in the mountains, or even the person's own bedroom. Some individuals will prefer a solitary scene, while others will prefer the presence of a trusted companion.

Assume a comfortable position in a quiet room, where you are not likely to be disturbed during your practice. Now prepare to begin your visualization, by relaxing yourself in body and mind. Release any emotional baggage of the day. Allow your muscles to become loose and limp. Guide your breathing to become slow, gentle, and relaxed. If it is comfortable, close your eyes, as this is conducive to visualization and imagination.

If you are distracted, bring your attention back to your special, peaceful place. Accept whatever restlessness is there and return to relaxation. You need not try hard to relax. At this moment, your only effort is to set aside effort.

In your mind's eye, visit your calm place. Use all your senses to experience it fully. See it in your mind's eye, notice the colors, the degree of light, and the shapes of your surroundings. Experience the sounds. Notice whether there is warmth or coolness, and whether there is a fragrance. Is there anything in this place that you can feel and experience through touch? Allow the full sensory presence of the place to wash over you.

Experience whether there is an emotional feeling to this place: Is it peaceful and soothing, and can you experience that peace in yourself? Is there a joyfulness, a happiness or a comic aspect to it? Can you experience the positive feeling of this place?

Or is there a sadness or sense of loss in this place? Can you experience this sadness or painful emotion with acceptance, as a part of you and your life?

Allow yourself to fully experience the sensory presence of this place and its emotional atmosphere. Stay with the image and the full experience. Soak it up, savour it, enjoy it and store it in your memory as an experience you can return to in the future.

Practical guidelines

Once you have fully experienced your selected place in a positive and soothing way, you can return to this place at any time and recover the sense of calm and tranquillity – or the sense of joy, sadness, loss or acceptance.

Experiment with selecting several different places and notice what emotional atmosphere is supported by each one. When you have identified two or more scenes that work well for you, evoking emotions and feelings that suit your purpose, then return to these same places intermittently, deepening your experience each time by using all your senses.

Occasionally, an individual will experience that a specific place that was initially peaceful and comforting becomes less welcoming or even threatening in some fashion. Consider the nature of this change and relate it to any traumatic experiences in your earlier life. You may wish to identify a new calm place that seems distinct from that past trauma. If new images repeatedly become threatening, it may be better to choose a different self-care exercise, such as progressive muscle relaxation or mindful breathing. If you have a counselor, this problem may provide a valuable topic for discussion.

Skill Module 4: Expressive writing

Journal writing is a simple tool for stress management and emotional wellness. Writing about your life and your feelings has positive effects on physical and emotional health. Extensive research by Dr James Pennebaker shows that individuals who write about their emotions and thoughts experience several benefits: increased feelings of wellbeing, reduced medical visits, reduced absenteeism from work, improved academic grades, and enhanced immune system functions. A study in the *Journal of the American Medical Association* showed that patients who wrote in a journal for three consecutive days showed improvements that were verified by their doctors. Arthritis patients showed reductions in arthritis symptoms, and people with asthma showed measurable improvements in breathing (Smyth *et al*, 1999).

Instructions

Obtain a blank notebook or diary. Commit yourself to writing regularly for 10 to 20 minutes several times per week. Each time you write in your journal, express your deepest thoughts and feelings about some important emotional event or issue that has affected you. In your writing, let go and explore your deepest emotions and thoughts. You might tie your topic to your relationships with others, including parents, lovers, friends, or relatives. Or you might tie it to your past, your present, or your future; or to who you have been, who you are now, or who you would like to be.

You may write about the same general issues or experiences each time you journal, or you may write about different topics each day. Your writings are personal and belong only to you. It is your decision and your decision alone to share your journal with another person. Some people will wish to share their journaling with a trusted friend or counselor. However, you will write more freely if you have no worries about a spouse or other person's reactions to what you write.

Do not worry about spelling, sentence structure, or grammar. There is no right or correct journal entry. Whatever you express in your journal today is your truth for this moment.

Initially, regular journaling – about three to four times per week – is valuable for acquiring the skill and the habit. Later, you may use journaling as a coping strategy. When you experience stress or begin to ruminate on a problem, take out your journal and begin to write. Remember, though, to set a length of time that is comfortable for you, anywhere from 10 to 20 minutes. Then continue writing until the time is up. When the time is up, stop, put away your journal, and resume your everyday activities. Sometimes, an individual will continue writing for hours and trigger unnecessary grief and emotional distress.

You do not need to write every day. Instead, think of expressive writing as a way to clarify your thoughts and emotions. This method is particularly powerful in helping you to get through emotional upheavals.

Practical guidelines

Many people are hesitant to write for fear of others discovering and reading their journal. Feel free to dispose of your writings after you have written the day's entry. No one need ever see what you have written. The process of self-expression is beneficial even if the text is immediately shredded, burned, or otherwise destroyed.

Resources

Lepore, S. J., & Smyth, J. M. (Eds.). (2002). *The Writing Cure: How expressive writing promotes health and emotional well-being.* American Psychological Association.

Pennebaker, J., & Evans, J. (2014). *Expressive Writing: Words that heal.* Idyll Arbor.

Smyth, J. M., Stone, A. A., Hurewitz, A., & Kaell, A. (1999). Effects of writing about stressful experiences on symptom reduction in patients with asthma or rheumatoid arthritis: A randomized trial. *Journal of the American Medical Association,* **281**, 1304-1309.

Skill Module 5: Mantra meditation

Meditation is one of the oldest disciplines for focusing attention and gaining control over the mind. For the most part, meditative techniques began as tools to help human beings achieve a greater spiritual awareness – a spiritual union with God, or with a spiritual dimension. Yet today, many people use meditation to produce relaxation, greater calmness, and relief from many forms of distress and illness. It is a practical form of self-care.

There are many kinds of meditation, ranging from concentrative meditation, in which the meditator full absorbs his or her consciousness in a single focus, such as a mantra, a candle, or the sunset, to an awareness meditation in which the meditator releases all focus, and mindfully accepts whatever enters the field of consciousness.

This exercise introduces a beginner's level mantra meditation. Mantra meditations are simple, requiring only that the meditator: 1) select a mantra – a sound, word, or phrase, 2) repeat or chant that mantra over and over, and 3) focus awareness fully on the mantra. This procedure helps many beginners to focus better, because the mantra seems to channel attention away from distractions.

Instructions

For this exercise, you will begin by choosing a word, syllable, or phrase that you experience as soothing and positive. Traditionally, meditative mantras came from Vedic or Buddhist sacred texts, such as the familiar "Om Shanti Om" ("Bless us with peace") or "Om Mani Padmé Hum" ("Hail the jewel in the lotus").

You may choose a non-religious word or phrase such as "One", "Peace", "Relax", or "Let it be". You may also choose a phrase from any religious or spiritual tradition. A Catholic might chant "Jesus, Mary, and Joseph", a Protestant might chant "The Lord is my Shepherd", a Jew might chant "Shalom" ("peace"), and a Muslim might chant "Inshallah" ("God willing" or "Allah willing").

1. Once you have selected a mantra, choose a quiet environment, with subdued lighting, where you are not likely to be disturbed. Set a clock or timer for a length of time comfortable for you – initially around 15 minutes, and longer when you are more experienced.

Appendix A: Instructions for self-care skills

2. Now assume a comfortable position, sitting on a mat or in a chair. Adjust your posture so you can sit comfortably for an extended period. Keep your spinal column straight, while allowing the rest of your body to relax. A stable posture grounds us and centres us, in mind and body.
3. Consciously release any baggage of the day – any problems, burdens, or anxieties. Release any physical tensions in your body as well. For this moment in time, allow yourself a period of respite from any need to address problems. Release these tensions and open yourself to this meditative experience.
4. If you wish, you may set an intention for your meditation, for example, "May this meditation bring me peace of mind amid my struggles", or "May this meditation help me find patience with my co-workers".
5. Close your eyes now if this is comfortable for you.
6. Begin to breathe slowly, gently, comfortably, and allow your breathing to relax your body and quiet your mind.
7. Now begin to gently repeat your mantra, either mentally or aloud. Repeating the mantra aloud may assist you to release distractions.
8. Wrap your awareness more and more around the feel and sound of the mantra.
9. Some meditators like to time the mantra with their breathing, inhaling and then chanting with the outbreath. "Inhale, mantra, inhale, mantra, …"
10. Should any distraction arise, simply notice it mindfully, accept it, and return your attention to the mantra and its repetition. If you repeatedly encounter distracting thoughts, try chanting the mantra aloud, and increase the volume moderately to focus your attention.
11. Accept this experience, however it unfolds. There is no right or wrong meditative experience, only the experience of this moment.
12. Allow your chanting of the mantra to become more and more automatic, until you can begin to feel that you are an observer, hearing and experiencing the mantra as if from a distance. At the same time, allow yourself to experience that you are in the mantra, that it surrounds you.
13. Enjoy the meditative experience as it continues to absorb you.
14. Continue chanting the mantra, adjusting your physical posture as needed, continuing to breathe slowly, gently, smoothly, without effort.
15. When your timer signals that your meditation session is ending, allow yourself an additional minute to slow the mantra, slow your breathing,

and store away memories of this experience. You can return to this experience later, when you have a few moments, simply by recalling these closing moments of the meditation.

16. Now stretch, relax, and rejoin your daily routines, carrying a more peaceful quality into your day.

Practical guidelines

1. Most individuals find it helpful to establish a routine with a daily practice time and a regular place or places for meditation. When possible, decorate your meditation space with spiritual paintings, inspirational posters, flowers, and spiritual symbols.
2. Experiment with varying your posture until you find a position that works well for you to keep you centred and awake. An upright posture is usually better than reclining, as reclining is conducive to sleep.
3. Be aware of cultivating a "beginners mind" each time you practice meditation, that is, an openness to experience whatever presents itself, no matter how knowledgeable you are from past education and training. Zen tradition includes the story of a master telling his student, "You are like this teacup, so full that nothing more can be added. Come back to me when the cup is empty." That is, empty your cup and become open to this new experience of meditation.
4. Choose a style and technique of meditation that works for you, with your temperament and preferences. However, we also encourage you to try out and learn several forms of meditation. Different techniques may help you better at various times, depending on your mood, stress level, and current life situation.
5. Appendix B provides links to several YouTube videos in which Donald Moss introduces other forms of meditation.

Skill Module 6: Mindfulness training

Mindfulness, acceptance, and compassion are words heard with increasing frequency as forms of self-care and coping. Mindfulness calls for the individual to develop a moment-to-moment awareness of present events, characterized by non-judging, non-striving, acceptance, non-attachment, trust, patience, and a beginner's mind (Kabat-Zinn, 2005). The Vietnamese Buddhist teacher, author and activist Thich Nhat Hanh described the goal of mindfulness as "…keeping one's consciousness alive to the present reality" (Hanh, 1976, p. 11).

Embracing mindfulness leads to a new and different approach to negative experiences. For example, the approach of mindfulness to anxiety and worry differs greatly from what is called cognitive therapy. Cognitive therapy encourages a person to dispute or confront irrational or negative thoughts, and to seek to restructure one's automatic thought processes. In contrast, mindfulness calls for the individual to observe the anxious thoughts and accept them, without any judgment or effort to change them.

Instructions

The following instructions encourage adopting a prevailing attitude of mindful awareness and acceptance. Mindfulness means "paying attention in a particular way: on purpose, in the present moment, and non-judgmentally" (Kabat-Zinn, 2005, p. 4). To begin learning mindfulness, choose a life situation that you know you will be entering in the near future. Review the guidelines here, and rehearse in your mind enacting these guidelines in the situation. Then, when you enter the situation, implement your mindfulness guidelines.

1. Be aware of noticing what is happening in this situation, as it unfolds.
2. Consciously suspend any judgment or critical thoughts about what happens, and accept your emotional response to the situation.
3. Be aware that it is not your responsibility to change anything that happens, anything that comes into your awareness, or your own inner response to this situation.
4. Trust that you will be able to perceive what is happening and accept whatever emerges, and that this acceptance is the optimal response.

5. Consciously accept what happens; accept this situation as it unfolds.
6. Be aware of letting go of all efforts to change this situation, and of letting go of all need to pass judgment on the situation or on yourself.
7. Be aware of your breathing while in this situation. Allow your breathing to slow and become gentle and relaxed. This enhances your ability to accept the events around you. If you find yourself struggling against the situation, turn your attention to the process of your breathing. Follow each in-breath into your body and each outbreath as it leaves your body. With each outbreath, whisper to yourself the word "accept".

Now leave the situation and review the various ways in which you were able to accept the situation mindfully. Avoid judging any inadequacies in your mindful coping. Rather, look for further extensions of the mindful acceptance that you would like to implement next time you enter the situation or other challenging situations.

You may carry the mindfulness guidelines everywhere you go in your daily life. Allow yourself to increasingly view the events of your life at a slight distance, through the lens of mindful awareness.

Resources

Hanh, T. N. (1976). *Miracle of Mindfulness*. Beacon.

Kabat-Zinn, J. (2005). *Wherever You Go There You Are: Mindfulness meditation in everyday life* (10th edition). Hachette Books.

Skill Module 7: Informal mindfulness meditation

In contrast to formal meditation, in which time is set aside to "practice", informal mindfulness meditation can be done during many common daily activities. Eating and walking are among the most frequent opportunities for a person to meditate. Instead of eating quickly without paying attention to the appearance or even the taste of the food (mindless eating), mindful meditative eating involves paying attention to all aspects of the food. Apply all of the principles of mindfulness to this snack or meal. Be fully present in this moment, allowing yourself to notice each aspect of the sensory experience of the food and of your body's response to eating. Accept the experience mindfully, without judging the experience or yourself.

The enjoyment of eating is greatly enhanced by noticing the colors, smell, taste, texture, and temperature of the food. Slowing down eating usually also decreases the amount of food that the person consumes, because the signals of fullness have enough time to reach the brain!

Another example is mindful meditative walking. The person notices everything in the immediate environment, but also pays attention to the noise their shoes make on the ground, the temperature of the air, the feeling of the breeze or sun on their face. Be fully present in this moment with the walking, with your body's movement, with the surroundings.

The same principle can be applied to exercise performed indoors, although it may be more difficult to maintain the mindful focus on the movement due to competing noises or interruptions.

In summary, instead of mindlessly rushing through activities, slow down and appreciate the movement, sensations, sights, sounds and smells found in your daily life. Be present in this moment, accepting it and enjoying it fully.

Resources

Birtwell, K., Williams, K., van Marwijk, H., Armitage, C. J., & Sheffield, D. (2019). An exploration of formal and informal mindfulness practice and associations with wellbeing. *Mindfulness*, **10**(1), 89-99. https://doi.org/10.1007/s12671-018-0951-y

Giannou, K., & Mantzios, M. (2023). Meditative and non-meditative mindfulness-based interventions for mind and body. *BMC Complementary Medicine and Therapies*, **23**, 235. https://doi.org/10.1186/s12906-023-04069-7

Appendix A: Instructions for self-care skills

Skill Module 8: Special mindfulness exercise

Embracing mindfulness leads to a new and different approach to negative experiences. The following exercise helps you develop a mindful attitude toward everyday life.

Instructions

This exercise provides a visualization portraying a vivid personal experience of mindful acceptance. Read these words, visualizing them as if you are present in the scene. Then enact them for your daily living.

1. Picture yourself on a train, passing across a landscape. Simply notice and accept what comes into view and passes from your awareness.
2. If landscape features come into view, you are not responsible for changing them, keeping them in view, or making them disappear.
3. If human beings come into view, engaged in activities, you are not responsible for judging their actions, solving their problems, keeping them in view, or making them disappear.
4. You may simply mindfully observe what comes into view and accept when each landscape feature or person passes from view.
5. Enjoy this ever-changing process of manifestation, as the images and events outside your window continue to change.
6. Now, carry the train window with you into your everyday life. Be aware of everything that happens as if you were on that train, observing through the window.

Practical guidelines

You may carry this mindfulness train window everywhere you go in your daily life. Allow yourself to increasingly view the events of your life through the glass of the train window, from the vantage point of a train passing through a landscape.

Be aware of experiencing a loving compassion for the people you view through the window of the train. You need not change these individuals; you need not argue with their words and actions. Allow yourself to see their struggles, while exercising acceptance and compassion for them as human beings, struggling through this same life.

Skill Module 9: Progressive muscle relaxation

Progressive muscle relaxation (PMR) was developed by Edmond Jacobson (1888-1983), a Harvard-educated physician and psychologist. Jacobson learned that most human beings can experience relief from tension and anxiety by learning a simple self-guided procedure.

In PMR, the individual alternately tenses and relaxes each muscle group throughout the body and pays close attention to the feelings and sensations during each moment of tension or relaxation.

This procedure increases both awareness and control: awareness of the subjective sensations accompanying both tension and relaxation and the contrast between the two, and a heightened control over muscle tension. With practice, many patients discover that they are more aware of the subtle onset of tension in everyday life, and begin to recognize specific stressors that are triggering muscular tension. The following instructions present a brief version of PMR.

Instructions

Assume a comfortable position in a quiet room. This exercise will guide you to relax each part of your body, progressively, from the feet all the way up to your head. Your breathing should be smooth, gentle, and relaxed. With each breath, inhale and fill your lungs with air, as if you were gently filling up a balloon. Then exhale, gently emptying your lungs, and notice the release of tension.

1. In a comfortable reclining position, close your eyes and take three slow, full breaths.
2. Bring your attention to your right foot. Bend your right foot upward at the ankle, pointing the toes toward your head. Hold this tension and position. Observe the tensions along the front of the lower leg and the stretching in the calf. Notice the difference between the tensing and the stretching. Now slowly release all tension and allow the foot to relax. Feel the contrasting sensations with relaxation.
3. Now bend your foot down, pointing the toes away from the body. Hold this position and observe the patterns of tension. Now slowly

Appendix A: Instructions for self-care skills

release the tension and again allow the leg and foot to relax. Feel the sensations of relaxation.
4. Contract your lower right leg toward your buttocks. Hold this position and feel the patterns of tension. Now slowly release all tension, position your leg comfortably, and become aware of the sensations accompanying relaxation.
5. Now extend your lower right leg, so that your upper and lower leg point outward and upward, away from your body. Feel the patterns of tension in the leg and anywhere else in the body. Slowly release all tension, returning your leg to rest. Feel the sensations of relaxation.
6. Repeat each of these actions on the left side of the body. Each time, sense the tensions as the muscle groups tighten, slowly release tension, and then enjoy the contrasting sensations accompanying relaxation.
7. Extend your right arm upward and extend your hand upward. Tense the right arm and hand and hold the tension. Be aware of the sensations of tension in the arm, and anywhere else in the body. Exhale and drop the arm. Roll the right arm from side to side, limbering the muscles. Now repeat with the left arm and hand.
8. Now contract the buttocks and inhale. Tighten your buttocks, hold your breath, and notice the increasing tension. Hold the tension a moment and slowly release. As the tension leaves your buttocks, exhale fully and study the sensations of relaxation. As you tense and relax each area of the body, notice the contrast between muscle tension and muscle relaxation.
9. Bring the shoulder blades together in the back. Squeeze tightly. Now release the shoulders and allow your entire upper body to become limp. Study the sensations of relaxation.
10. Bring both shoulders up to your ears. Hold them up. Now exhale and allow them to sag. Now push the shoulders downward. Hold that tension briefly. Now release and allow your upper body to become limp.
11. Tighten the facial muscles. Make your face like a prune. Squeeze more tightly. Now exhale and release tension.
12. Roll the neck gently from side to side, limbering the muscles.

Practical guidelines

1. Practice several times a day, at home and in work settings. You can practice the *tense-hold-relax* sequence in any setting, gently tensing in a fashion not noticeable for others, and it will assist you in relaxing your musculature in that moment.
2. Progressive muscle relaxation serves two purposes. First, you will increase your *awareness* of any muscle tension in your body. This means you will begin to notice the onset of tension before it becomes severe. Second, you will learn to *relax* the muscles. You will finally learn to relax immediately each time your body reacts to life stress.
3. You can repeat the *tense-hold-relax* sequence with any muscle group thoughout the body to enhance a fuller relaxation. For example, there are several muscles around the eyes which frequently tense as a person thinks intently. Tensing and releasing those muscles reduces the facial tensions associated with worry.
4. If any steps in this progressive muscle relaxation exercise trigger muscle cramps, either tense the muscles more gently, or move to another form of relaxation.
5. Additional, more detailed progressive muscle relaxation exercises are available (Davis *et al*, 2019).

Once you have learned to tense the muscles in several areas of the body, and can then switch off tensions to near zero, it is important to practice and apply the new skills in everyday life. First, commit yourself to practice several times a day, at home and in work settings. For example, consider setting the goal to practice PMR each time you stop at a traffic light, or each time you face the bathroom mirror. Secondly, become aware of tension in the muscles, throughout the course of everyday life. Finally, use these new skills to reduce physiological tension and emotional tension in stressful situations, whenever they occur.

Resources

Davis, M., Eshelman, E. R., & McKay, M. (2019). *The Relaxation and Stress Reduction Workbook* (7th edition). New Harbinger Publications.

Skill Module 10: Self-hypnosis

Hypnosis is a technique in which a trained professional assists subjects in experiencing changes in their sensations, perceptions, thoughts, feelings, and behaviors. Once in hypnosis, subjects usually experience a different state of mind, with focused attention and a calm, relaxed, pleasant kind of experience. In the hypnotic state, most people find they are better able to modify behavior, lifestyle, and emotions.

Self-hypnosis is a process in which individuals guide themselves into a hypnotic state, without the assistance of a hypnotist.

The following exercise provides written instructions to achieve a hypnotic state on your own, allowing you to relax, deepen your confidence and hope about your situation, and enhance your overall wellbeing. This exercise involves straining your eyes upward, and then moving down a staircase into a deeper and deeper state of hypnotic relaxation.

Read through the exercise several times, until you can proceed through it with only an occasional glance at the instructions.

Instructions

1. Assume a comfortable position, either seated or reclining.
2. Release any tensions or pressures of the day, allowing your body to relax and your mind to quieten.
3. Now look directly ahead at the wall in front of you.
4. While keeping your head stationary, allow your eyes to drift upward, to the point where they are moderately strained.
5. Choose a place there, and keep your eyes straining upward, fixed on that same spot on the wall ahead and above.
6. Notice the deepening heaviness and fatigue in your eyelids. They become heavier and heavier and more and more fatigued, as you strain to continue looking upward.
7. At some point, you may find yourself blinking more and more frequently, or you may not blink at all. You may find a growing urge to allow the eyes to sink and close.
8. Eventually, you will allow the eyes to close, no longer resisting the heaviness and fatigue in the eyes and eyelids. Your eyes may close entirely on their own, or you may finally decide to allow them to close.

9. Now experience what a relief it is, as your eyes close and remain closed, and you drift into a deeper and deeper state of hypnotic relaxation.
10. Rest gently for a moment, enjoying the ease and deepening relaxation as you continue drifting deeper and deeper into hypnosis.
11. Now, when you feel ready, visualize in your mind a marble staircase take shape before you, a staircase leading you downward into an even deeper hypnotic state.
12. Grasp the solid wooden banister and prepare to go down one step at a time, counting with each step. One, stepping down and going into a deeper state of relaxation.
13. Continue downward in your mind. Two, down, down, deeper and deeper. Three, four, stepping down and experiencing yourself more and more relaxed, mind and body relaxed. Five, six, down, down, deeper and deeper. Seven, eight, you can begin to see a comfortable place at the foot of the stairs, an inviting and comfortable place. Nine, ten, stepping down, down, and finally you reach the bottom, and discover a comfortable peaceful place and an inviting seat at the base of the stairs.
14. Allow yourself to take a seat and now simply allow yourself to experience a profoundly comfortable and relaxed state, your body more and more fully relaxed and your mind peaceful, quiet, so deeply relaxed.
15. Allow yourself to enjoy this deep hypnotic relaxation and this comfortable place. You may see the surroundings and details in your mind, seeing the sights and hearing the sounds. This place invites you to relax more and more fully, absorbing its serenity.
16. Enjoy this experience and consciously store it away, save it, as something you can return to and fully re-live whenever you have free time to seat yourself or recline, fixate your eyes, and once again descend the staircase.
17. When you feel ready to bring this time of relaxation and renewal to an end, allow yourself to rise up from this seat. In your mind, turn toward the staircase again and grasp the banister. Begin to re-trace your steps upward now, counting from ten to one, at your own pace.
18. Notice that you experience yourself gradually once again becoming more alert, returning to an everyday state of mind. As you count down towards one, allow your eyes to gradually open, and look around your actual physical surroundings in the room where you began.
19. Stretch, limber your body, and orient yourself to the present moment.

20. Notice, however, that you continue to carry that deepened state of relaxation in your body and in your mind. You may feel aspects of it surging up in you in the days to come, often when you least expect it.

Practical guidelines

Some people naturally respond more deeply to hypnosis, and others less so. Whatever your response to the instructions, it is right for you. You can assess whether this exercise brings you sufficient benefit to use it regularly.

Repeating this exercise several times a week will make it more automatic. You may come to find that you can simply think of going into a hypnotic state and it will begin to happen, without the detailed steps of the exercise.

Appendix B:
Apps, YouTube videos, books, audio recordings, and websites for self-care and lifestyle change

Apps

This section lists some of the leading apps providing self-regulation-oriented guidance.

Aptiva – The Aptiva app provides guidance for exercise and fitness. https://aaptiv.com/

Evia – Evia has downloadable apps for hot flashes, night sweats, insomnia, and other symptoms of menopause. The developer is Gary Elkins, a leader in hypnosis research and practice, in conjunction with MindsetHealth. www.eviamenopause.com/

Fooducate – Fooducate provides an app to guide better food choices and enhance overall nutrition. www.fooducate.com/

Headspace – Headspace provides downloadable apps for meditation, sleep enhancement, stress management, and other issues. Headspace has a multi-disciplinary staff and faculty. www.headspace.com/

HealthTap – HealthTap provides physician-led online medical visits, as well as guidance to address diabetes, hypertension, headache and a variety of other health problems. www.healthtap.com/

Nerva – Nerva provides guidelines for hypnotic exercises designed to moderate symptoms of irritable bowel syndrome and gastrointestinal distress. Michael Yapko, Gary Elkins, and Irving Kirsch, leaders in the hypnosis field, form the scientific advisory board. https://try.nervaibs.com/

Noom – Noom has downloadable apps for weight management and dietary change. Noom uses a coaching approach to assist nutritional change. www.noom.com/

Reveri – Reveri has downloadable apps providing self-hypnosis for improved sleep, stress reduction, habit change, enhanced attention, enhanced exercise, and dietary change. The chief scientific officer is David Spiegel, a leading hypnosis researcher. www.reveri.com/

Sleep Cycle – Sleep Cycle provides a free basic app and a paid premium subscription, designed to enhance sleep quality and remediate a variety of specific sleep problems. www.sleepcycle.com/

WaterLlama – The WaterLlama app aids the individual in tracking hydration on a daily basis. https://waterllama.com/

WW – WW, formerly known as Weight Watchers, provides an app providing live coaching, guidance for grocery shopping, and tracking for foods. www.weightwatchers.com/us/how-it-works/ww-app

YouTube videos

The following YouTube videos were recorded by Donald Moss, and are available on YouTube individually and on the Saybrook University self-care website (www.youtube.com/@saybrookuniversityself-car5910).

For each meditation, enter the accompanying URL (weblink) into your computer browser to access the resource.

Breath meditation: This 15-minute exercise guides you to use your own breathing as the basis for meditation. Breathing gently and slowly can be transformative emotionally and spiritually.
www.youtube.com/watch?v =_FXeH2aykOs&t = 149s

Autogenic training: Autogenic training mobilizes our innate ability for healing and recuperation. AT consists of a series of simple, easily learned mental exercises which link mind and body together in association with deep relaxation.
www.youtube.com/watch?v = EIyBu9R-9n4

Calm scene: This 15-minute meditation introduces a familiar guided imagery technique: the calm scene. Each participant will choose their own safe and quiet place and absorb themselves in its sense of peace and calm.
www.youtube.com/watch?v =_NGhCgYiEiw&t = 160s

Mantra meditation: This 15-minute meditation exercise uses a mantra, a word or phrase gently to guide you into a meditative state.
www.youtube.com/watch?v = vgf6iWA2-_s&t = 34s

Progressive muscle relaxation: This 15-minute webinar introduces progressive muscle relaxation, a technique that highlights the difference between relaxed and tense muscles, and develops a differential awareness of muscle tension and a corresponding ability to release tensions. This is a wonderful self-care technique, and is widely used by counselors, coaches, and healthcare providers to manage tension and relieve pain.
www.youtube.com/watch?v = C90aZJo1GY0&t = 216s

Meditation on letting go: This 15-minute meditation encourages the personal development of letting go, detaching from the hustle and bustle of life, and re-discovering both serenity and direction.
www.youtube.com/watch?v = wnuPzN-pKqQ&t = 32s

Meditation on nature: This 15-minute guided nature meditation invites you to use your own imagination to immerse yourself in nature. In nature, we find personal restoration and renewal.
www.youtube.com/watch?v = TczyJqbfq-I&t = 239s

Meditation on self-love: This 15-minute meditation guides the listener to cultivate and deepen love and compassion for oneself.
www.youtube.com/watch?app = desktop&v = ZaN7R0pqXck

Books

The following books provide guidance for self-care and lifestyle change for your health and wellness. They are available from Amazon and elsewhere.

Anderson, B. (2020). *Stretching: 40th anniversary edition*. Shelter Publications.

Boone, M. S., Gregg, J., & Coyne, L. W. (2020). *Stop Avoiding Stuff: Twenty-five microskills to face your fears and do it anyway*. New Harbinger.

Borges, A. (2019). *The More or Less Definitive Guide to Self-Care*. The Experiment.

Bourne, E. (2000). *Healing Fear: New approaches to overcoming anxiety*. MJF Books.

Burdick, D. (2013). *Mindfulness Skills Workbook for Clinicians and Clients*. PESI Publications and Media.

Childre, D., Martin, H., & Beech D. (2011). *The HeartMath Solution* (reprint edition). HarperOne.

Davis, M., Eshelman, E. R., & McKay, M. (2019). *The Relaxation and Stress Reduction Workbook* (7th edition). New Harbinger Publications.

Eifert, G., & Forsyth, J. (2016). *The Mindfulness and Acceptance Workbook for Anxiety: A guide to breaking free from anxiety, phobias, and worry using acceptance and commitment therapy* (2nd edition). New Harbinger Publications.

Frates, B., Tollefson, M., & Comander, A. (2021). *Paving the Path to Wellness Workbook*. Healthy Learning.

Goldstein, E., & Stahl,. B. (2015). *MBSR Every Day: Daily practices from the heart of mindfulness-based stress reduction*. New Harbinger Publications.

Gordon, J. (2009). Unstuck: Your guide to the seven-stage journey out of depression. Penguin Books.

Gros, D. F. (2021). *Overcoming Avoidance Workbook: Break the cycle of isolation and avoidant behaviors to reclaim your life from anxiety, depression or PTSD*. New Harbinger.

Hanh, T. N. (1976). *Miracle of Mindfulness*. Beacon.

Hanson, R. (2016). *Hardwiring Happiness: The new brain science of contentment, calm, and confidence* (reprint edition). Harmony Books.

Harris, R. (2022). *The Happiness Trap: How to stop struggling and start living* (2nd edition). Shambhala.

Kabat-Zinn, J. (2005). *Wherever You Go, There You Are: Mindfulness meditation in everyday life* (10th edition). Hachette Books.

Kabat-Zinn, J. (2013). *Full Catastrophe Living: Using the wisdom of your body and mind to face stress, pain, and illness* (revised edition). Bantam.

Kalb, R., Giesser, B., & Costello, K. (2012). Multiple Sclerosis for Dummies. John Wiley and Sons.

Katz, R., & Edelson, M. (2017). *Cancer Fighting Kitchen: Nourishing, big flavor recipes for cancer treatment and recovery* (2nd edition). Ten Speed Press.

Khazan, I. Z. (2019). *Biofeedback and Mindfulness in Everyday Life: Practical solutions for improving your health and performance*. W. W. Norton.

Kushner, H. S. (2004). *When Bad Things Happen to Good People* (reprint edition). Anchor Books.

LaDyne, R. (2020). *The Mind-Body Stress Reset: Somatic practices to reduce overwhelm and increase well-being*. New Harbinger Publications.

Lagos, L. (2020). *Heart, Breath, Mind: Train your heart to conquer stress and achieve success*. Houghton Mifflin.

Lepore, S. J., & Smyth, J. M. (Eds.). (2002). *The Writing Cure: How expressive writing promotes health and emotional well-being*. American Psychological Association.

Lorig, K., Sobel, D., Laurent, D., Minor, M., Gonzalez, V., & Gecht-Silver, M. (2020). *Living a Healthy Life with Chronic Conditions: Self-management skills for heart disease, arthritis, diabetes, depression, asthma, bronchitis, emphysema, and other physical and mental health conditions* (5th edition). Bull Publishing Company.

Macedo, D. (2021). *The Sleep Fix: Practical, proven, and surprising solutions for insomnia, snoring, shift work, and more*. William Morrow.

McGonigal, K. (2016). *The Upside of Stress: Why stress is good for you and how to get good at it* (reprint edition). Avery.

McGrady, A., & Moss, D. (2013). *Pathways to Illness, Pathways to Health.* Springer.

McGrady, A., & Moss, D. (2018). *Integrative Pathways: Navigating chronic illness with a mind-body-spirit approach.* Springer.

McKay, M., Fanning, P., Pool, E., & Zurita Ona, P. E. (2022). *Healing Emotional Pain Workbook.* New Harbinger.

Millman, M. P., & Kermott, C. A. (2020). *Mayo Clinic Guide to Self-Care.* Mayo Clinic Press.

Nass, T., Freeman, J., & Rodgers, A. B. (2020). *Lupus: A patient care guide for nurses and other health professionals.* Diane Publishing Company.

Nestor, J. (2020). *Breath: The new science of a lost art.* Riverhead Books.

Ornish, D. (1996). *Dr Dean Ornish's Program for Reversing Heart Disease.* New York, NY: Ivy Books/Ballantine Books.

Pennebaker, J., & Evans, J. F. (2014). *Expressive Writing: Words that heal.* Idyll Arbor, Inc.

Potter-Efron, R. (2012). *Healing the Angry Brain.* New Harbinger Publications.

Prochaska, J. O., & Prochaska, J. M. (2016). *Changing to Thrive: Using the stages of change to overcome the top threats to your health and happiness.* Hazelden Publishing.

Rosmarin, D. H. (2023). *Thriving with Anxiety: Nine tools to make your anxiety work for you.* Harper Horizon.

Stahl, B., & Goldstein, E. (2019). *A Mindfulness-based Stress Reduction Workbook* (2nd edition). New Harbinger Publications.

Starlanyl, D., & Copeland, M. E. (2001). *Fibromyalgia and Chronic Myofascial Pain: A survival manual.* New Harbinger Publications.

Unger, T. Borghi, C., Charchar, F., et al. (2020). International Society of Hypertension global hypertension practice guidelines. *Journal of Hypertension*, **38**(6), 984-1004.

Walker, M. (2018). *Why We Sleep: Unpacking the power of sleep and dreams* (reprint edition). Scribner.

Williams, F. (2018). *The Nature Fix*. W. W. Norton.

Audio recordings

The following audio recordings are available as CDs, audiobooks, or MP3 audio downloads. I have provided a website where each recording can be ordered.

Kabat-Zinn, J. (2002a). *Guided mindfulness meditation* (series 1). (Audio CD). Better Listening LLC. www.soundstrue.com/

Kabat-Zinn, J. (2002b). *Guided mindfulness meditation* (series 2). (Audio CD). Better Listening LLC. www.soundstrue.com/

Kabat-Zinn, J. (2006). *Mindfulness for beginners: Reclaiming the present moment.* (Audiobook). Sounds True. www.audible.com/

Kornfield, J. (2010). *Meditation for beginners.* (Audiobook). Sounds True. www.soundstrue.com/

Naparstek, B. (2000). *A guided meditation for healthful sleep.* (Audio CD/MP3). Hay House. www.healthjourneys.com/

Naparstek, B. (2009). *A meditation to support a healthy immune system.* (AudioMP3). Hay House. www.healthjourneys.com/audio-library

Naparstek, B. (2007). *Guided meditations to help with anxiety and panic.* (Audio CD). Health Journeys. www.healthjourneys.com/

Naparstek, B. (2010). *A meditation to help you with radiation therapy.* (Audio MP3). Health Journeys. www.healthjourneys.com/audio-library

Naparstek, B. (2022a). *A meditation to help you fight cancer.* (Audio MP3). Hay House. www.healthjourneys.com/audio-library

Naparstek, B. (2022b). *A guided meditation to help you manage diabetes.* (Audio CD/MP3). Hay House. www.healthjourneys.com/

Weil, A., & Kabat-Zinn, J. (2006). *The Andrew Weil audio collection.* (Audiobook). Sounds True. www.soundstrue.com/

Appendix B: Apps, YouTube videos, books, audio recordings, and websites for self-care and lifestyle change

Websites

This section lists useful websites for health and wellness.

American College of Lifestyle Medicine. (no date). Lifestyle medicine for all: Interventions for treating chronic disease in under-resourced patient populations. https://lifestylemedicine.org/articles/lifestyle-medicine-for-all/ (accessed September 2024)

American Heart Association. (2024). Heart attacks and stroke symptoms. www.heart.org

American Heart Association. (2023). Managing blood pressure with a heart-healthy diet. Health Topics. www.heart.org/en/health-topics/high-blood-pressure/changes-you-can-make-to-manage-high-blood-pressure/managing-blood-pressure-with-a-heart-healthy-diet (accessed September 2024)

American Heart Association. (2024). High blood pressure. Health Topics. www.heart.org/en/health-topics/high-blood-pressure (accessed September 2024)

American Psychological Association (APA). (2009). An action plan for self-care. www.apaservices.org/practice/good-practice/Spring09-SelfCare.pdf (accessed September 2024)

American Psychological Association (APA). (2019). Depression treatment for adults. www.apa.org/depression-guideline/adults#:~:text=Adults%20generally%20receive%20three%20to,treatment%20of%20depression%20in%20adults (accessed September 2024)

American Psychological Association. (2023). 11 healthy ways to handle life's stressors. www.apa.org/topics/stress/tips (accessed September 2024)

American Psychological Association. (2023). Stress effects on the body. www.apa.org/topics/stress/body (accessed September 2024)

Anxiety and Depression Association of America. (2023). What are anxiety and depression. www.adaa.org

Arthritis Foundation. (no date). About arthritis. www.arthritis.org/about-arthritis (accessed September 2024)

Arthritis Foundation. (no date). Nine exercises to help hand arthritis. www.arthritis.org/health-wellness/healthy-living/physical-activity/other-activities/9-exercises-to-help-hand-arthritis (accessed September 2024)

Association of Behavioral and Cognitive Therapy. (2023). Fact sheets of ABCT. www.abct.org/fact-sheets/ (accessed September 2024)

Bergquist, S. H. (2016). How stress affects your body. (YouTube). TED-Ed. www.youtube.com/watch?v = v-t1Z5-oPtU

Brain and Spine Foundation. (no date). Migraines. www.brainandspine.org.uk/health-information/fact-sheets/migraine/ (accessed September 2024)

CDC. (2024). Arthritis in adults age 18 and older: United States, 2022. National Center for Health Statistics. Centers for Disease Control and Prevention. https://www.cdc.gov/nchs/products/databriefs/db497.htm#:~:text = Data%20from%20National%20Health%20Interview,those%20age%2075%20and%20older. (accessed February 2025)

Cleveland Clinic. (2020). Emotional stress: Warning signs, management, when to get help. https://my.clevelandclinic.org/health/articles/6406-emotional-stress-warning-signs-management-when-to-get-help (accessed September 2024)

Cleveland Clinic (2022). How exercise helps lower blood pressure and eight activities to try. Health Essentials. https://health.clevelandclinic.org/exercises-to-lower-blood-pressure (accessed September 2024)

Cleveland Clinic (2022). Six types of foods that lower blood pressure. Health Essentials. https://health.clevelandclinic.org/foods-to-lower-blood-pressure (accessed September 2024)

Cleveland Clinic (2022). Conversion disorder. https://my.clevelandclinic.org/health/diseases/17975-conversion-disorder (accessed September 2024)

Cleveland Clinic. (2024). Insomnia. https://my.clevelandclinic.org/health/diseases/12119-insomnia (accessed September 2024)

Cleveland Clinic. (2024). Tension headaches. https://my.clevelandclinic.org/health/diseases/8257-tension-headaches (accessed September 2024)

Davis, B. (2020). Stress response. Billings Clinic. (YouTube). www.youtube.com/watch?v = oE9DNlpXpaI (accessed September 2024)

Diabetes UK. (2024). Diabetes: The basics. (2-minute video). www.diabetes.org.uk/diabetes-the-basics (accessed September 2024)

Gillette, H. (2022). How to stop using avoidance as a coping method: Five ways. Psych Central website. https://psychcentral.com/health/how-to-stop-avoiding-what-scares-or-overwhelms-you#why-is-it-unhelpful (accessed September 2024)

Harvard Health. (2024). Recognizing and easing the physical symptoms of anxiety. www.health.harvard.edu/mind-and-mood/recognizing-and-easing-the-physical-symptoms-of-anxiety

HeartMath Institute (2021). emWave Pro®. https://store.heartmath.org/emWave-PC/emwave-pro.html (accessed September 2024)

Johns Hopkins Medicine. (2023). Diabetes self-management patient education material. (Free informational booklets and handouts). www.hopkinsmedicine.org/general-internal-medicine/core-resources/patient-handouts (accessed September 2024)

Kets deVries, M. F. R. K. (2009). Six steps to overcome shame. Insead. https://knowledge.insead.edu/leadership-organisations/six-steps-overcome-shame (accessed September 2024)

Learning about Diabetes. (2021). About diabetes. (Free informational booklets.) https://learningaboutdiabetes.org/programs-consumer/ (accessed September 2024)

Levi, A. (2023). What is the DASH diet? Health Newsletters. www.health.com/dash-diet-7972360 (accessed September 2024)

Lincolnshire Partnership NHS Foundation Trust. (2022). Exploring mindfulness and the 5-4-3-2-1 grounding activity. www.lpft.nhs.uk/young-people/lincolnshire/about-us/whats-new/grounding-activity (accessed September 2024)

Mayo Clinic. (2022a). Depression (major depressive disorder). www.mayoclinic.org/diseases-conditions/depression/symptoms-causes/syc-20356007 (accessed September 2024)

Mayo Clinic. (2022b). Functional neurologic disorder/conversion disorder. www.mayoclinic.org › syc-20355197

Mayo Clinic Health System. (2024). Specialty care made personal. www.mayoclinichealthsystem.org (accessed September 2024)

Mayo Clinic Staff. (2024). DASH diet: Healthy eating to lower your blood pressure. Nutrition and Healthy Eating. Mayo Clinic. www.mayoclinic.org/healthy-lifestyle/nutrition-and-healthy-eating/in-depth/dash-diet/art-20048456 (accessed September 2024)

Mind Infoline. (2024). Post-traumatic stress disorder. www.mind.org.uk/information-support/types-of-mental-health-problems/post-traumatic-stress-disorder-ptsd-and-complex-ptsd/self-care/ (accessed September 2024)

Mind Infoline. (2024). Stress. www.mind.org.uk/information-support/types-of-mental-health-problems/stress/signs-and-symptoms-of-stress/ (accessed September 2024)

National Alliance on Mental Illness (NAMI). (2017). Depression. www.nami.org/About-Mental-Illness/Mental-Health-Conditions/Depression

National Alliance on Mental Illness. (2024). Who we are. www.nami.org/About-NAMI/Who-We-Are/ (accessed September 2024)

National Center for Complementary and Integrative Health. (2024). Relaxation techniques: What you need to know. https://nccih.nih.gov/health/relaxation-techniques-what-you-need-to-know (accessed September 2024)

National Health Service, United Kingdom. (2022). Treatment: Generalized anxiety disorder in adults. www.nhs.uk/mental-health/conditions/generalised-anxiety-disorder/treatment/ (accessed September 2024)

National Headache Foundation. (2024). Our vision: A world without headache. https://headaches.org/ (accessed September 2024)

National Institute of Diabetes and Digestive and Kidney Diseases. (2023). What is diabetes? www.niddk.nih.gov/health-information/diabetes/overview/what-is-diabetes (accessed September 2024)

National Institute of Mental Health. (2023). Mental health medications. www.nimh.nih.gov/health/topics/mental-health-medications

Appendix B: Apps, YouTube videos, books, audio recordings, and websites for self-care and lifestyle change

National Institute of Mental Health (NIMH). (2023). Depression. www.nimh.nih.gov/health/topics/depression

National Institute of Neurological Disorders and Stroke. (2024). Brain basics: Understanding sleep. www.ninds.nih.gov/health-information/public-education/brain-basics/brain-basics-understanding-sleep (accessed September 2024)

National Institutes of Health. (no date). DASH eating plan. www.nhlbi.nih.gov/education/dash-eating-plan

Pfizer (2024). Treating migraine attacks: Breaking down migraine treatments. www.nurtec.com/how-to-treat-migraines#preventive (accessed September 2024)

PsychCentral. (2022). Letting go of the past: Why it's so hard to get rid of painful memories. https://psychcentral.com/health/letting-go-of-the-past-why-memories-remain-painful-over-time (accessed September 2024)

PsychCentral. (2022). Seven self-care tips for PTSD, https://psychcentral.com/ptsd/ptsd-self-help#grounding (accessed September 2024)

PsychCentral. (2022). What is trauma? https://psychcentral.com/health/what-is-trauma#symptoms (accessed September 2024)

Psychology Today. (2023). Self-care: All things to all people? www.psychologytoday.com/us/blog/changepower/202308/self-care-all-things-to-all-people (accessed September 2024)

Psychology Tools. (2022). Post-traumatic stress disorder, www.psychologytools.com/self-help/post-traumatic-stress-disorder-ptsd/ (accessed September 2024)

Self-Help Toons. (no date). Mindfulness and our breath. (YouTube). www.youtube.com/watch?v=4Ma0oMofy8U (accessed September 2024)

Sleep Station. (2024). Sleep stages: What are they and why are they important. www.sleepstation.org.uk/articles/sleep-science/sleep-stages/ (accessed September 2024)

Taylor, M. (2021). Adult coloring book: Seven benefits of coloring. WebMD. www.webmd.com

The Royal Institution. (2017). The science of stress: From psychology to physiology. (YouTube). www.youtube.com/watch?v=uOzFAzCDr2o (accessed September 2024)

Twill. (no date). Why mindfulness is a superpower: An animation. (YouTube). https://youtu.be/w6T02g5hnT4?si=iX2zjlSlBAkaMRMo (accessed September 2024)

Vemu, P. L., Yang, E., & Ebinger, J. (2024, February). 2023 ESH hypertension guideline update: Bringing us closer together across the pond. American College of Cardiology. www.acc.org/latest-in-cardiology/articles/2024/02/05/11/43/2023-esh-hypertension-guideline-update (accessed September 2024)

Web MD. (2017). How to treat a tension headache. www.webmd.com/migraines-headaches/features/treatments-tension (accessed September 2024)

Web MD. (2024). What is migraine. www.webmd.com/migraines-headaches/migraines-headaches-migraines (accessed September 2024)

WebMD. (2024). Anxiety and panic disorders guide: Treatment. www.webmd.com/anxiety-panic/guide-chapter-anxiety-panic-treatment (accessed September 2024)

World Health Organization. (2024). Migraine and other headache disorders. www.who.int/news-room/fact-sheets/detail/headache-disorders (accessed September 2024)

Appendix C:
Healing Pathways Worksheets

This appendix provides Healing Pathways Worksheets, designed to increase your awareness of the emotional impact of living with illness, and to help you design activities to enhance your quality of life.

Healing Pathways Worksheet, Chapter 4:

Regaining control and making decisions on health habits

The first recommendation made to a patient newly diagnosed with Type 2 diabetes is to start a diet diary, then be prepared to make changes in diet. The diabetes educator highlights specific changes in amount, type, and timing of meals. As described in Chapter 4, the changes can be overwhelming to a patient and their family. Remember that food is much more than just calories. Food consumption is a social experience – it can bond people together, or it can separate them. Choices of food and preparation of specific dishes are strongly influenced by culture, ethnicity, and environment.

Principles of healthy eating apply to all adults, so this worksheet was designed for anyone needing to or wanting to change their eating habits. We recommend the reader consult the references at the end of this worksheet to find details of nutritional plans that consider food sensitivities, allergies, or illness related limitations in food choices.

Adult eating is actually driven by habits which were formed during development in the environment of family, caregivers and peers. Think back to your early years and answer the questions below:

Was there enough food?	yes / no
What was the quality of food?	good / poor
Were meals a social event?	yes / no
Did you sit at a table or on a tray in front of the television?	table / tray
Were you on screens while you are eating?	yes / sometimes / no
Was food used as a reinforcer for good behavior or as a punishment for bad behavior?	yes / no

Appendix C: Healing Pathways Worksheet, Chapter 4: Regaining control and making decisions on health habits

Next, consider how your experiences influenced your current eating habits. What traditions have you kept, and what have you changed?

Which of the traditions is the most important to you?

There are many models, guidelines and instructions for what a healthy diet should be for adults. You may see "catchy" terms such as "eat the rainbow", which refers to selecting fruits and vegetables with a variety of colors. There are also recommendations for the timing of meals. For example, always eat breakfast, avoid large meals within three hours of bedtime, and four to five small meals are healthier than two large meals per day. However, we warn the reader that searching the topic "timing of meals" can lead to more confusion, because you will see descriptions of fasting schedules in addition to the basic timing described above.

Many people try to read all the instructions and then give up before they even start to make actual changes. Or they attempt too much change at once and become overwhelmed. In addition, drastic changes to the composition of family meals may be rebuffed by partners, children or parents.

Fortunately, the most common models for good nutrition share many concepts: decrease consumption of sugar in beverages and in foods; increase consumption of vegetables and fruits; limit alcohol use; decrease foods high in saturated fats; decrease red meat; and increase whole grains. One example of a model is called "My Plate". It divides a typical plate into four quadrants. Half of the plate should be fruits and vegetables, a quarter of the plate should be whole grains, and one-quarter should be protein. Dairy is represented by the shape of the bottom of a glass or cup.

Review your current eating habits. Which are not healthy when you consider the recommendations of "My Plate"? When are you most likely to eat high-calorie foods or eat large quantities of food?

_____

_____

When do you eat even though you are not hungry?

_____

_____

Do you feel pressure from peers or from family members to eat more or less of culturally sanctioned foods? Which foods and which people?

_____

_____

In Chapter 4, Louisa snacked before bedtime and when she awoke during the night. She changed that habit by eating smaller amounts or lower calorie foods. In time, she only had a few crackers before bed and a glass of water during the night. Louisa realized that her food choices were strongly influenced by her family and her culture. Tradition and family created strong pressure to continue to eat large calorie-laden meals. Her next habit change was to choose healthier foods when she was alone and not under the influence of her husband – which was at breakfast time.

Let's put your eating patterns, culture, and current state of health into one picture.

Consider the smallest step or change that you can make in your diet. Do not attempt major changes or many changes at the same time. Do not attempt major changes that affect the entire family. One small success lays the foundation for larger successes. In addition, your mind must habituate (get used) to the change in nutrition just as your body adjusts to finding the taste of sweetness in fruit instead of chocolate cake. If, as a child, you were not sure that there would be a dinner that night, seeing a smaller plate of food may trigger anxiety. Reprograming your mind with a different message is an important part of eating a healthier diet. For example, enjoying the taste of salty snacks is a conditioned response of mind and body. Decreasing salt intake initially makes food taste bland and boring. In time, however, you will come to appreciate the actual taste of the food and find heavily salted foods unappetizing.

Describe the change that you will make today or tomorrow.

Continue each day. Missing a day does not mean you should give up or that you will never improve your diet. Resume the healthy change and keep trying.

In summary, each small successful change lays the foundation for bigger successes. Over time, each success becomes normal for your body and your mind. If visible to others, the change becomes normal to them also. Then you move on to the next goal and the process repeats.

Additional reading

Duhigg, C. (2014). The Power of Habit: Why we do what we do in life and business. Random House.

Frates, B., Tollefson, M., & Comander, A. (2021). Paving the Path to Wellness Workbook. (Chapter 8: Nutrition). Healthy Learning.

Useful websites

American College of Lifestyle Medicine. (2024). Food as medicine. https://lifestylemedicine.org/nutrition-as-medicine/ (accessed September 2024)

Diabetes UK. (no date). Eating with diabetes. www.diabetes.org.uk/guide-to-diabetes/enjoy-food/eating-with-diabetes (accessed September 2024)

Mayo Clinic. (2024). Diabetes diet: Creating your healthy eating plan. www.mayoclinic.org/diseases-conditions/diabetes/in-depth/diabetes-diet/art-20044295 (accessed September 2024)

USDA My Plate. (2024). Healthy eating for adults. www.myplate.gov/tip-sheet/healthy-eating-adults (accessed September 2024)

Healing Pathways Worksheet, Chapter 5:
Heredity is not destiny

Many people with a family history of cancer or heart disease feel a sense of pessimism about their future. It is often challenging to believe that their own self-care or lifestyle changes can make a difference, when several relatives have died young with similar health problems. They often believe something like "Heredity is destiny".

Do you have serious health problems in your family history? List the relatives who had serious health problems and what those problems were:

1. _____
2. _____
3. _____
4. _____

Did any of these relatives die young or suffer serious disability because of their illness? List here the relative's name, and their age when they began to suffer disability or their age when they died:

1. _____
2. _____
3. _____

As we mentioned in Chapter 2, a medical researcher named Dean Ornish showed very clearly how new self-care practices and lifestyle modifications could improve the health of patients who already suffered from serious heart disease. In his treatment programs, patients learned to meditate, practiced yoga, mastered basic stress-management skills, increased their activity levels, and modified their everyday diets.

The patients in Ornish's treatment program lowered their blood pressure, reduced their triglyceride and cholesterol levels, and in some cases restored blood flow to arteries that had been obstructed. Many also showed reduced anxiety and increased positive mood.

Following the Pathways Model, you can make similar changes in your everyday lifestyle, learn some new self-care practices such as meditation, and improve your overall health. This same approach can be applied to heart disease, diabetes, chronic pain, anxiety, depression, and many other long-term conditions.

We cannot erase heredity, but we can moderate its impact! If many members of your family have had high cholesterol and high blood pressure, for example, then you may be at risk for these same problems. But making positive lifestyle changes can greatly reduce that risk!

What are some self-care practices that appeal to you? How ready are you to begin using them or increase your frequency of using them?

1. _____
2. _____
3. _____
4. _____

What are some lifestyle changes that you believe would benefit your health condition? Are you ready to begin making these changes?

1. _____
2. _____
3. _____
4. _____

Now choose the simplest self-care practice and the simplest lifestyle change from your two lists above. Make a commitment on the line below. Start today to make those changes.

I will ... _____
_____

Remember that results do not occur quickly and are often not dramatic.

Keep track of the changes that you are making. At the end of the first week, assess your progress and write about it on the line below.

During the past week I ... _____

_____

Continue to increase self-care and lifestyle changes, moving on from the easiest change to the next easiest one, and so on. Review these changes with your health coach, your healthcare provider, or your change buddy.

Healing Pathways Worksheet, Chapter 6:
Assessing your engagement with nature

Viewing nature is believed to rest the brain and reduce the effects of stress on your body and mind. Being immersed in a natural setting reduces anxiety and improves mood, reduces blood pressure, and enhances immune function. After time outdoors, you may find that you are more mentally attentive and can concentrate better than before you went outside.

Research shows that even exposure to indoor plants has positive effects for your physical health and emotional wellbeing. Living in greener neighbourhoods compared to residing in an urban environment is associated with better health, better emotional health, and a longer lifespan, as are gardening or maintaining living green plants in the home.

The *Forest Bathing* movement advocates planning regular immersion in nature for the health and wellbeing effects on anyone who participates.

What types of nature and nature-oriented activities do you enjoy?

What is your favourite season of the year?

When you left the house this morning, what do you remember seeing?

We are often on autopilot, rushing out of the house, not seeing anything and getting to work and not remembering how we got there. How often do you let yourself pause and focus on something in nature? Daily? Weekly? Monthly? Only on holiday?

Wherever you are reading this, get up and look outside. Concentrate on one tree, flower, hill, bank, pond, or lake. Breathe slowly and absorb the view. Let yourself feel the calming effects of this nature experience.

There are certain aspects of nature that you can experience every day. Others require a drive, or a flight to a resort. Resolve to view and appreciate one thing from nature every day. You may want to keep a diary of these experiences and refer back to them when you have been stuck in the house – perhaps due to bad weather or illness.

Consider your readiness and set one or two nature-focused goals that you believe you are ready to implement.

Initial nature-based goals:

1. _____

_____

2. _____

_____

Additional resources

Buzzell, L., & Chalquist, C. (Eds.). (2009). *Ecotherapy: Healing with nature in mind.* Counterpoint.

Clifford, M. A. (2018). *Your Guide to Forest Bathing: Experience the healing power of nature.* Red Wheel.

Plotkin, B. (2008). *Nature and the Human Soul: Cultivating wholeness and community in a fragmented world.* New World Library.

Williams, F. (2017). *The Nature Fix: Why nature makes us happier, healthier, and more creative.* W. W. Norton.

Wohlleben, P., & Billinghurst, J. (2022). *Forest Walking: Discovering the trees and woodlands of North America.* Greystone Books.

Healing Pathways Worksheet, Chapter 7:
Transforming perceptions of stress

Building cognitive skills

This worksheet is a guide designed to help you to first become aware of, and then change, your attitudes towards and perceptions of stress. How you react to stress depends on three factors: 1. your assessment of the type of stress (positive, negative or neutral); 2. the intensity of the stressful situation (mild, moderate, severe, expected or a surprise, familiar to you or new); and 3. your belief in your ability to manage or control the stress (low ability, uncertain about your ability, or high competence).

Consider the example below:

> Five people win tickets to an amusement park. Two are thrilled, one has been there before and is not interested, one gets sick on rides so refuses the tickets, and one is terrified at the thought of going.
>
> Five people have the same opportunity, but their reactions differ widely, depending on how each person perceives the situation, their past history with amusement parks, and their biological make up.

Think of a situation from your life and describe your reaction and that of others who were with you. _____

_____

_____

_____

_____

_____

When you have experienced a major stress reaction, remember that the event itself did not cause your *alarm* or *fear* reaction. It is our perception of events that actually causes our tense muscles, anger, sadness, joy, or happiness. How we perceive a situation leads to our self-talk (what we say to ourselves about the situation). Types of self-talk include positive, negative, neutral, encouraging, critical, wary, fearful, and instructional (the mind telling the body what to do and how to do it). In turn, self-talk guides our feelings and our reactions.

Consider the example below of what you could experience on your way home from school or work.

Stimulus:	Self-talk:	Reaction or response:
A few minutes delay at a traffic light.	This doesn't matter; I'm not in a hurry.	Ignore it.
Sounds of a fire engine.	This is important.	Pay attention and pull over to the side.
Seeing that the trees have changed color.	The trees are beautiful.	Enjoy the view and relax.
Dangerous road conditions.	I could skid.	Slow down.

Next, consider different perceptions of the same stimuli and notice how the self-talk changes and the reactions are different.

Stimulus:	Self-talk:	Reaction or response:
Delay at a traffic light.	I will be late for work; I should have left earlier.	Upset stomach.
Sounds of a fire engine.	What if they are going to my house?	Fear and tense muscles.
Seeing that the trees have changed color.	Winter is coming. I hate winter.	Sad and tearful.
Dangerous road conditions.	I don't need to slow down; nothing will happen.	Inattention, feeling of superiority; skidding.

Now, work on how to change or counter your negative, catastrophic self-talk. Consider the examples below and indicate your typical response.

Example 1: You are given a difficult task at work. Your automatic self-talk is *"I can't do it"*. What is the best counter thought from the list below?

   a. I must block this thought.
   b. I am not smart enough to complete this task.
   c. Having the thought means that I really can't do it; thoughts are reality.
   d. It's hopeless.
   e. I am aware of the thought; it is not based on fact. I will try to do the task.

Thoughts are not reality; they may or may not be accurate. "Hopeless" and "not smart enough" are judgments, not facts. Blocking the thought only makes it disappear for a few seconds. Acknowledge the thought, change your perception of the task and decide to try.

Example 2: You are asked to give a short presentation at your job. Your automatic self-talk is *"Don't get nervous"*. What is the best action to take?

   a. Spend time around other nervous people.
   b. Repeat: *don' t get nervous, don't get nervous.*
   c. When it is your turn to present, talk really fast to get it over with.
   d. Be aware of the nervousness and slow your breathing.

Repetition of the word "nervous" intensifies the experience of being nervous. The anxiety of others can increase your own anxiety; don't seek out other nervous people. If you have worked hard on the presentation, getting it over with will not feel good. Practice the presentation to decide on the pacing. We recommend you become aware of your nervousness so that you can take appropriate action to relax.

Example 3: You are a student. Your tutor announces that the next chapter and the next exam are going to be the hardest in the whole course. Your automatic self-talk may be: *"The next few weeks are going to be a nightmare"*, or *"I found the earlier chapters hard to learn so I will be hopeless at the new chapter"*. What is the best cognitive coping strategy?

   a. I am not even going to try.
   b. I have got this far; I can complete the hard chapter if I work at it.
   c. I am mad at the teacher for giving us this hard chapter.
   d. I should drop out of this class.

You are already in the class so someone believes that you can succeed! You can't control the sequence of chapters in the book, but you can be appreciative of the warning of the upcoming difficult chapter. If you perceive the warning as a benefit instead of a threat, your attitude towards the work will change. You can control the amount of effort that you give to the chapter.

For the next week, pay attention and be aware of your self-talk. Note how you feel when you are saying negative, unrealistic words to yourself.

Write down some examples:

Self-talk   **Feeling**
_____   _____
_____   _____
_____   _____
_____   _____

You can use your mental skills to decrease overreactions. Stop perceiving neutral events as completely negative and build a positive mindset over time. Learn to be realistic, not fatalistic, about actual stressful events. Differentiate between things that you have control over and those that you don't. Know how to tell the difference. Practice countering your negative self-talk with more realistic assessments of situations and your own abilities.

In Chapter 7, Angela experienced a return of her headaches after many years of good control. Her work hours changed and resulted in changes in sleep, eating and social schedules. Angela took full blame for the relapse; she was self-critical and hard on herself. She talked about the headaches being her fault, that she had brought them on herself. She put herself into a forced choice situation: job or romantic relationship. Her thoughts of failure led to muscle tension and anxiety; her anxiety prevented her from getting enough sleep. Tension and fatigue cycled back to more negative thoughts; it became a vicious cycle. Angela learned the importance of perception and self-talk; she worked on reframing situations so that she looked at them differently. Ultimately, she regained her self-confidence.

References

McGonigal, K. (2016). *The Upside of Stress: Why stress is good for you and how to get good at it* (reprint edition). Avery.

Healing Pathways Worksheet, Chapter 8:
Overcoming embarrassment, shame, and isolation

Many patients experience embarrassment and shame over their physical symptoms, and over uncontrollable mood swings triggered by their long-term health condition. Not being able to make plans ahead of time can be hard on relationships, leading to both shame and isolation. Over time, many patients with long-term conditions lose contact with once-close friends. Even family members may withdraw in the face of cancelled plans and unpredictable mood swings.

Relationships are key to healing shame and embarrassment. Disclosing one's sense of shame to others and identifying behaviors and life changes that embarrass you can reduce the shame and increase self-acceptance.

Your relationship with yourself is important, too. Are you ready to forgive yourself for having your long-term health condition?

Do you have any negative thoughts that increase your self-blame? Some Christians believe that God is punishing them with the illness for past mistakes. Yet Christians believe that God is loving, and this doesn't seem very loving! A Hindu patient with chronic pain blamed *bad karma* for his condition, based on some act of unkindness in his past or in a previous life. Remember that illness is a universal part of life, affecting good people and bad alike, without any reason!

What aspects of your condition trigger embarrassment, shame, and isolation?

_____

_____

Are there moments when you feel much more self-acceptance?

_____

_____

Appendix C: Healing Pathways Worksheet, Chapter 8: Overcoming embarrassment, shame, and isolation

Do you have any negative thoughts that seem to build self-blame and shame, and interfere with self-acceptance?

_____

_____

Do you feel more isolated now than before the onset of your condition?

_____

_____

Which relationships bring you the greatest sense of loss and distress?

_____

_____

Are there people in your life that you still feel comfortable spending time with?

_____

_____

How often do you feel distress over embarrassment, shame, or isolation? Daily? Weekly? Monthly? Hardly ever?

_____

_____

While reading this, take a mental inventory of your most important relationships, including family, friends, and colleagues. Make a list of these individuals:

_____

_____

_____

_____

Make an additional list of small steps you feel ready to take to restore contact with these people:

1. _____
2. _____
3. _____
4. _____

Are there embarrassing things about your condition and your current life that you feel ready to risk sharing with any of these contacts? List the item to share and the person here:

1. _____
2. _____
3. _____
4. _____

Additional resources

Kets deVries, M. F. R. K. (2009). *Six Steps to Overcome Shame*. Insead. https://knowledge.insead.edu/leadership-organisations/six-steps-overcome-shame (accessed September 2024)

McKay, M., Fanning, P., Pool, E., & Zurita Ona, P. E. (2022). *Healing Emotional Pain Workbook*. New Harbinger.

Healing Pathways Worksheet, Chapter 9:

Overcoming avoidance behaviors and recovering a rewarding life

Many long-term conditions and illnesses are accompanied by pain or anxiety. All too often, people who experience pain begin to avoid activities that trigger it. In some ways, this is common sense. If a stove is hot, don't touch it. If it hurts to walk, don't walk. Unfortunately, avoidance often backfires and worsens one's suffering. People who avoid physical activity suffer muscle deconditioning, and then it takes even less activity to trigger pain.

Similarly, people who experience anxiety and fear begin to avoid situations and activities that trigger these emotions. If public or crowded places seem to trigger panic attacks, then avoid crowded supermarkets, and so on. But anxiety and fear tend to generalize over time. Initially, supermarkets might seem anxiety provoking at busy times, but over time the supermarket may seem frightening at any time and even small convenience stores may begin to seem intimidating.

Many people with pain or anxiety end up with very narrow lives. Unfortunately, when human beings narrow their lives to avoid pain and distress, their lives feel empty. Having a diminished life can trigger a sense of loss and depressed mood.

Let's take an initial inventory.

How often do you find yourself engaged in actively avoiding some situation that might trigger distress, pain, or anxiety?

Daily? Weekly? Monthly? Hardly ever?

Now take a few minutes, and list below some of the activities and situations that you have begun to avoid or limit, since you began to suffer pain and distress.

1. _____
2. _____
3. _____
4. _____
5. _____

Are you feeling distressed or upset about the loss of some of these activities? Are you finding yourself depressed and yearning for the life you used to enjoy? While reading this, take a mental inventory of your most important pastimes and activities, the ones that contribute most to making your life worth living.

Which of these activities do you most wish to recover?

1. _____
2. _____
3. _____
4. _____

Can you think of strategies that might help you in moving toward some recovery of these activities? Or could you modify the activities, so that you could enjoy them with less distress? For example, exercising gently in a warm-water pool – called aquatherapy – often enables people with arthritis or long-term myofascial pain to better tolerate exercise. Similarly, some yoga teachers offer gentle yoga or chair yoga classes, for people who cannot tolerate aggressive muscle stretching.

Appendix C: Healing Pathways Worksheet, Chapter 9:
Overcoming avoidance behaviors and recovering a rewarding life

List possible strategies or approaches to taking back some of your past favourite activities:

1. _____

2. _____

3. _____

4. _____

Make an additional list of small steps you feel ready to take to overcome avoidance and reclaim places and activities in your life:

1. _____

2. _____

3. _____

4. _____

Additional resources

Boone, M. S., Gregg, J., & Coyne, L. W. (2020). *Stop Avoiding Stuff: Twenty-five microskills to face your fears and do it anyway*. New Harbinger.

Gillette, H. (2022). *How to Stop Using Avoidance as a Coping Method: Five ways*. Psych Central website. https://psychcentral.com/health/how-to-stop-avoiding-what-scares-or-overwhelms-you#why-is-it-unhelpful (accessed September 2024)

Gros, D. F. (2021). *Overcoming Avoidance Workbook: Break the cycle of isolation and avoidant behaviors to reclaim your life from anxiety, depression or PTSD*. New Harbinger.

Healing Pathways Worksheet, Chapter 10:
Mind and body in long-term health conditions

Long-term illness is a mind-body problem. Every long-term condition has strong medical and emotional elements. When human beings are depressed or anxious, they often develop headaches, stomach distress, elevated blood pressure and other physical symptoms.

Do you sometimes have physical symptoms at the same time that you have more stress in your life? Describe a recent time when this happened:

Does your doctor ever run tests for physical illness and the medical tests do not show any clear problems?

Are there certain negative emotions that occur over and over in your life? Describe them:

Sometimes physical symptoms are simple stress-related disorders. That is, our human stress response causes activation of our nervous system and hormone system, directly causing physical symptoms.

Relaxation skills, hypnosis, biofeedback, and guided imagery can all reduce the effects of stress on our bodies. What skills have you learned so far to relax your body?

Appendix C: Healing Pathways Worksheet, Chapter 10: Mind and body in long-term health conditions

Set a goal today to increase your practice of some kind of relaxation skill:

_____

_____

Other times, we suppress emotions, refuse to acknowledge them, and these emotions convert directly into physical symptoms that seem to speak for us. This is called "conversion disorder". Our body converts our emotional distress into physical symptoms.

Have you already identified some troublesome emotions that may be causing your distress? Name them:

_____

_____

Often, we can process troublesome emotions by discussing them at length with a therapist or close friend. Sometimes, writing about your feelings in a journal will also help. Use the lines below to start writing about a difficult or uncomfortable feeling:

1. _____

_____

2. _____

_____

Are you ready to set a goal about discussing, journaling, and exploring your negative emotions? Record a goal related to your emotions below:

_____

_____

Additional resources

American Psychological Association. (2023). 11 healthy ways to handle life's stressors. www.apa.org/topics/stress/tips (accessed September 2024)

Cleveland Clinic. (2020). Emotional Stress: Warning signs, management, when to get help. https://my.clevelandclinic.org/health/articles/6406-emotional-stress-warning-signs-management-when-to-get-help (accessed September 2024)

Cleveland Clinic (2022). Conversion disorder. https://my.clevelandclinic.org/health/diseases/17975-conversion-disorder (accessed September 2024)

Pennebaker, J., & Evans, J. F. (2014). *Expressive Writing: Words that heal*. Idyll Arbor, Inc.

Healing Pathways Worksheet, Chapter 11:
Mastering the terror of the unknown

Anxiety is an unpleasant experience of physical sensations in one or more parts of the body, mental and emotional distress, unpredictable behaviors and sometimes a spiritual crisis. Variety is the norm in anxiety disorders. Physical symptoms may be experienced in the heart, stomach, muscles or respiratory system. Mental signs of anxiety include difficulty focusing, distraction, self-doubt, rapid and scattered thoughts, and difficulty making decisions. Examples of emotional experiences are nervousness, fear and sometimes anger.

Some individuals' experience of anxiety is spiritual; they question their beliefs, turn away from their faith or, in contrast, believe that their faith will solve all their problems. Behaviorally, the anxious individual may move faster than usual, sleep less, sleep more, or may be inactive or frozen, unable to move towards or away from the stressor. Having multiple reactions to stress suggests that a variety of interventions can be effective – and indeed, this is true.

Identifying your anxiety reactions

On the lines below list at least one example of your usual anxiety reactions in each category.

Physical   Emotional

Cognitive/mental   Behavioral

Spiritual

Now identify your strongest (primary) and next strongest (secondary) anxiety responses.

Primary   Secondary

_____   _____

Next, identify your quickest (primary) stress response and your next quickest (secondary) stress response.

Primary   Secondary

_____   _____

Many people find that their body is their first response system, but not necessarily their strongest reaction. In survival situations, the body reacts seconds before any other system. Consider the example of touching a hot stove. Your arm moved before you said "ouch!" Similarly, a stomach cramp may occur as a stress response before you realize that you are afraid.

Awareness of that first reaction is important. Awareness leads to recognition, understanding, and eventual mastery. Your stress responses may be automatic if they have occurred many times before in the same or similar situations. Describe below a situation when you reacted without thinking and then later questioned your actions, because you realized that the response was not really necessary or was inappropriate.

_____

_____

_____

_____

_____

Introduce a pause

Pausing after our first awareness of anxiety gives the brain time to analyze the situation. Consider this sequence:

Stimulus → Awareness → PAUSE → Breathe → Think → Decide what to say and do

The PAUSE interrupts our automatic and impulsive rush into anxiety.

The best way to practice this skill is to anticipate a stressor that is likely to occur today or tomorrow. Imagine yourself in this situation and then visualize the sequence above. Repeat, repeat, repeat.

Energy management

The next section considers energy management strategies. Anxiety drains energy from the body, mind, and spirit. Tense muscles use energy, whether they are tightened because you are anxious or because you are riding your bike. Rapid, repetitive thoughts exhaust the ability to concentrate and focus. If worries keep you up at night and you are not rested in the morning, the lack of sleep intensifies your anxiety. This occurs because you believe that you are not physically strong enough, emotionally stable enough or cognitively sharp enough to manage the stress.

What are the times of day where you feel the most energetic?

_____

_____

And the least energetic?

_____

_____

When you plan your day, schedule your most demanding activities during your most energetic times of the day. When energy supplies are low, scheduling tasks and planning are important. In contrast, when you have plenty of energy, your planning does not have to be so specific and detailed, because there is excess energy and some can be wasted.

Use mindfulness skills (paying attention in the moment, without judgment) during your most difficult tasks. When you begin to feel anxious, pause, step back, and slow your breath or use progressive muscle relaxation for a few minutes. Then refocus on the task and keep on going. Counter negative, self-defeating thoughts. Don't try to fight or suppress the anxiety itself – accept it for the moment. Don't judge yourself harshly. Instead, change the self-talk from "I am anxious because I can't do it" to "I am feeling challenged because this is an important task". If you can anticipate the difficult task, even by an hour, activate the rehearsal and imagery strategies described above.

Additional reading

Loehr, J., & Schwartz, T. (2003). *The Power of Full Engagement: Managing energy, not time, is the key to high performance and personal renewal* (reprint edition). Free Press.

Useful websites

American Psychological Association. (2023). Stress effects on the body. www.apa.org/topics/stress/body (accessed September 2024)

Harvard Health. (2024). Recognizing and easing the physical symptoms of anxiety. www.health.harvard.edu/mind-and-mood/recognizing-and-easing-the-physical-symptoms-of-anxiety (accessed September 2024)

Mind Infoline. (2024). Stress. www.mind.org.uk/information-support/types-of-mental-health-problems/stress/signs-and-symptoms-of-stress/ (accessed September 2024)

Healing Pathways Worksheet, Chapter 12:

Integrating the past and living fully in the present – living with difficult memories

Trauma and the resulting long-term condition, post-traumatic stress disorder (PTSD) are the focus of Chapter 12. This worksheet takes a broader view. Individuals may experience psychological effects of memories that are not diagnostically labelled as trauma. To the person, however, the experience was disturbing; images of it return to their mind and sometimes impair function. Some examples might include:

- You were embarrassed when you spilled a red drink on your shirt in school and the other kids made fun of you.
- You were awkward during your first sexual encounter, and it didn't go well. You never wanted to see that person again, but you see her/him often in your dreams.
- On your first week in your new job, you made a significant error which came to the attention of the section chief. It wasn't your fault because you were instructed incorrectly by a peer. You always wonder if it was done on purpose or innocently. You blame yourself for not knowing.

These situations would not be encompassed by the formal definition of trauma, but to the person whose mind returns to the awkwardness, fear, or humiliation, the effects can be long term and damaging.

On the lines below, describe a troublesome memory.

_____

_____

_____

_____

It seems to the sufferer that these memories, generated by past events, refuse to stay in the past because difficult memories are triggered by current events. The person is taken by surprise, feeling invaded and out

Appendix C: Healing Pathways Worksheet, Chapter 12:
Integrating the past and living fully in the present – living with difficult memories

of control, even powerless to stop the images; it is difficult to clear one's mind from the memory. Emotions and behaviors follow the memory. The person may feel angry, sad, isolated and helpless. They may be irritable around others, or leave a social event abruptly.

On the lines below, describe the emotional, behavioral, and social effects of your difficult memory. If you have multiple difficult memories, choose the one that affects you *the least*, not the memory that creates the most vivid images and strongest reaction. Resolving difficult memories is a gradual process.

_____

_____

_____

_____

Next, list all the triggers that can elicit the memory, such as situations, people, words, smells, sounds, weather, crowds, isolation, being yelled at, or getting the silent treatment.

_____

_____

_____

Strategies for managing and eventually resolving difficult memories

Triggers: Anticipate the trigger if possible. Imagine yourself pausing when you are triggered so that you don't automatically react. Describe your effort to predict a trigger.

_____

_____

Decreasing the effect of the triggers: Ground yourself to the earth. The memory may try to take you back months or years. Resist that force and touch earth. Repeat the self-talk that you are not in the memory, you are in the present. Try that right now. Repeat: "I am not the memory; the memory is from the past; I am in the present. That same person, people, or situation does not exist in the present and cannot hurt me."

Use the *five things exercise* to ground yourself in the present.

What are five things that you can see? Four sounds that you can hear? Three things that you can touch? Two things that you can smell? One thing that you can feel with your fingers or on your skin?

Use the lines below to note what you see, hear, feel, taste and smell right now.

_____

_____

_____

Breathe in and out; breathe in calm and release tension with the exhale. You can control your breathing, and you can release your own tension.

Be grateful that you are no longer in that difficult time. Write three things that you are grateful or thankful for today.

_____

_____

_____

Use your cognitive skills – minimize self-blame, and be compassionate towards yourself as you would to a friend who is suffering. Write three statements of patience and compassion.

_____

_____

_____

Appendix C: Healing Pathways Worksheet, Chapter 12:
Integrating the past and living fully in the present – living with difficult memories

If you are comfortable with prayer, pray to your higher power for healing. Write a prayer on these lines:

_____

_____

_____

If you have acted badly (e.g., irritably, angrily, unreasonably) during your memory episode, apologize for these actions that occurred when you were triggered. Family and friends may not understand your words or actions and, feeling hurt or angry, may believe that they did something wrong. An apology prevents a cycle of aggravating people, their reactions, reinforcement of your bad behavior and so on from happening. Write an apology that you can use in a triggering situation.

_____

_____

_____

The above are ways to manage an existing situation. We also recommend these strategies as prevention tools for recurring difficult memories.

Develop resources for support: people that are close to you, internet support groups, in-person support groups. Regarding internet groups, ensure that there is a credentialed facilitator and that the approach is positive and encouraging. Be very cautious about the re-living of a traumatic memory with an internet support group.

Consider adopting a pet that can become part of your life. Pets are non-judgmental and they require care and commitment from their adult. A special bond often occurs between people and their pets, as described in Chapter 9. Animals can sense when their human is distressed, and they will provide comfort.

Do not allow hours of idle time. Develop activities that you enjoy; have a plan for each day. Isolation and boredom often open the mind to rumination, negativity, and recurrence of the memory.

Conclusion

In summary, resolution of traumatic or highly disturbing memories may require the assistance of a professional trained in trauma informed therapy. However, you can work towards acceptance and resolution as described above, and through that work regain a sense of control and peace.

Useful websites

Lincolnshire Partnership NHS Foundation Trust. (2022). Exploring mindfulness and the 5-4-3-2-1 grounding activity. www.lpft.nhs.uk/young-people/lincolnshire/about-us/whats-new/grounding-activity (accessed September 2024)

Mind Infoline. (2024). Post-traumatic stress disorder. www.mind.org.uk/information-support/types-of-mental-health-problems/post-traumatic-stress-disorder-ptsd-and-complex-ptsd/self-care/ (accessed February 2025)

PsychCentral. (2022). Letting go of the past: Why it's so hard to get rid of painful memories. https://psychcentral.com/health/letting-go-of-the-past-why-memories-remain-painful-over-time (accessed September 2024)

PsychCentral. (2022). Seven self-care tips for PTSD. https://psychcentral.com/ptsd/ptsd-self-help#grounding (accessed February 2025)

PsychCentral. (2022). What is trauma? https://psychcentral.com/health/what-is-trauma#symptoms (accessed September 2024)

Psychology Tools. (2022). Post-traumatic stress disorder. www.psychologytools.com/self-help/post-traumatic-stress-disorder-ptsd/ (accessed September 2024)

Self-Help Toons. (no date). Mindfulness and our breath. (YouTube). www.youtube.com/watch?v=4Ma0oMofy8U (accessed September 2024)

Twill. (no date). Why mindfulness is a superpower: An animation. (YouTube). https://youtu.be/w6T02g5hnT4?si=iX2zjlSlBAkaMRMo (accessed September 2024)